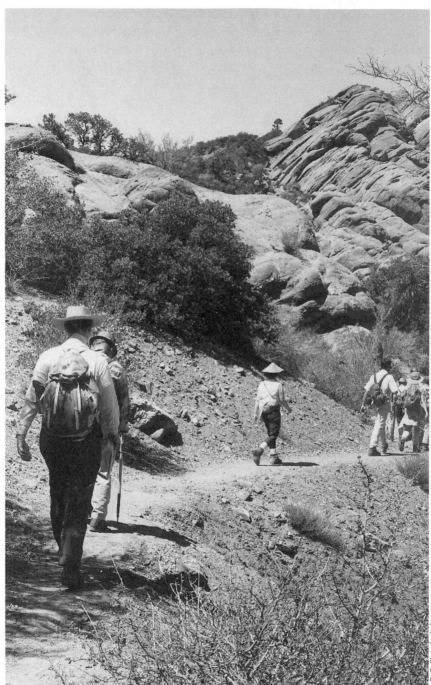

Trails of the
ANGELES

John W. Robinson
with Doug Christiansen

WILDERNESS PRESS ... *on the trail since 1967*

Trails of the Angeles: 100 Hikes in the San Gabriels

9th EDITION 2013
  2nd printing 2015

Copyright © 1971, 1973, 1976, 1979, 1984, 1990, 1998, 2005, 2013
  by John W. Robinson and Doug Christiansen

Front cover photo copyright © 2013 by Doug Christiansen
Interior photos, except where noted, by John W. Robinson
Pocket map design: Chris Salcedo/Blue Gecko, using data from John W. Robinson,
  Laurence Jones, Doug Christiansen, and U.S. Geological Survey topos
Cover design: Scott McGrew
Book design: Larry B. Van Dyke and Margaret Copeland/Terragraphics

ISBN: 978-0-89997-714-0

Manufactured in the United States of America

Published by: **Wilderness Press**
                Keen Communications
                P.O. Box 43673
                Birmingham, AL 35243
                800-443-7227; FAX 205-326-1012
                info@wildernesspress.com
                wildernesspress.com

Visit our website for a complete listing of our books and for ordering information.

Distributed by Publishers Group West

Cover photo: Near Oak Spring (Hike 7)

Frontispiece: Trail to Devil's Punchbowl (Hike 69)

Library of Congress Cataloging-in-Publication Data

Robinson, John W., 1929-
  Trails of the Angeles: 100 hikes in the San Gabriels / John W. Robinson with
  Doug Christiansen. — Ninth edition.
    pages cm
  ISBN 978-0-89997-714-0 — ISBN 0-89997-714-6
  1. Hiking—California—San Gabriel Mountains—Guidebooks. 2. San Gabriel
    Mountains (Calif.)—Guidebooks. I. Title.
  GV199.42.C22S277 2013
  917.94'93—dc23

                            2013013548

SAFETY NOTICE: Although Wilderness Press and the author have made every attempt
to ensure that the information in this book is accurate at press time, they are not
responsible for any loss, damage, injury, or inconvenience that may occur to anyone
while using this book. You are responsible for your own safety and health while in the
wilderness. The fact that a trail is described in this book does not mean that it will be
safe for you. Be aware that trail conditions can change from day to day. Always check
local conditions and know your own limitations.

Contents

Western End of the San Gabriels Hikes: Liebre–Sawmill–Sierra Pelona

HIKE

Front Range of the San Gabriels Hikes

HIKE

Backcountry Hikes: West Fork of the San Gabriel River to the Desert

HIKE

Middle High Country Hikes:
Above the North and East Forks of the San Gabriel River

Eastern High Country Hikes: Mount San Antonio to the Eastern End

HIKE

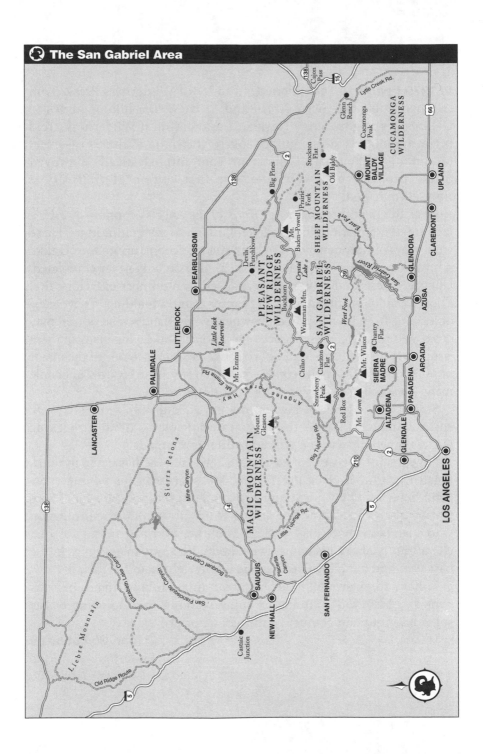

Preface to the Eighth Edition

In 1970 I wrote to Tom Winnett, founder of Wilderness Press. Tom had just published *Sierra North* and *Sierra South,* hiking guides to California's mighty Sierra Nevada. I asked Tom if Wilderness Press might be interested in a guidebook to the trails of the San Gabriel Mountains of Southern California. Tom enthusiastically approved of my project, and a year later, the first edition of *Trails of the Angeles* appeared.

Over the next three decades, *Trails of the Angeles* continued to be a favorite of Southern California hikers, much to my gratification. These were years of strenuous work to keep the guidebook up-to-date. Unlike a novel or most works of nonfiction, a guidebook is never completed. Change is constantly taking place, caused by a number of factors: fire, flood, abandoning of old trails and campgrounds, building of new ones, objections from private property owners whose land a road or trail may cross, and new US Forest Service regulations. Underlying many of these issues is the fact that the San Gabriels rise next door to one of the major population centers on the continent, which results in swarms of people using—and often overusing—these mountains.

Still, it was a labor of love on my part. Countless weekends were spent doing what I enjoy the most: tramping over old trails, checking out realigned or new ones, and meeting new friends.

Now, mainly because of advancing age, the time has come to relinquish work on *Trails of the Angeles.* My successor is a young, energetic hiker I met on the Mount Wilson Trail several years ago, Doug Christiansen of Sierra Madre. Doug is an airline pilot by profession who spends many of his free days rambling over the mountains that rise abruptly above his home. I've hiked with Doug many times in the past year and am convinced that he is the right man for the job.

I offer a fond farewell to my many mountain hiking friends of years gone by. May you continue to enjoy walking the footpaths of the splendid mountain country of the San Gabriels.

John W. Robinson
Fullerton, California
January 2005

Preface to the Ninth Edition

"Keeping a guidebook up-to-date is a never-ending job."
So wrote John W. Robinson many years ago in the preface to an early edition of *Trails of the Angeles*, and he has repeated the phrase often since. This has never been truer than in the seven years since the last edition was published. A series of natural and man-made disasters, culminating in the devastating 2009 Station Fire, have conspired to confound and frustrate hikers, nature lovers, and all who love the San Gabriel Mountains.

As a result, there have been many changes to the book. Several hikes—so noted in the text—are still off-limits due to the fire; others have only recently been reopened, and the repairing and reworking of trails is ongoing. These trail trips have been retained in the hope and expectation that nature—aided by the efforts of the US Forest Service and dedicated groups of volunteers—will slowly but surely restore what man has come so close to destroying. I have reluctantly removed and replaced four hikes in the book. Gone is the short stroll up Vetter Mountain and its historic lookout; the lookout burned to the ground in the Station Fire. The Bichota Canyon and Allison Gold Mine trails became so overgrown and eroded that these unsafe hikes have been replaced. Lastly, fire damage and persistent access problems at San Sevaine Flats led to the removal of that trail trip from the book.

In their place, I have chosen four excellent new hikes: two in the front range above Duarte and La Verne, a very scenic trail trip on the north side of the range from South Fork Campground to Vincent Gap, and a spectacular and challenging portion of the old North Backbone Trail on the back side of Mount Baldy, recently reintroduced after a multiyear absence from this guide.

Happily, there have been some positive developments in the past few years. Access roads to upper San Gabriel Canyon and Chantry Flat have finally been repaired. And two new wilderness areas were designated in the San Gabriels in 2009, protecting and preserving thousands of acres of vital habitat and watershed.

There is still much to see and explore, and much to enjoy and celebrate, in this fascinating mountain country.

Doug Christiansen
Pasadena, California
May 2013

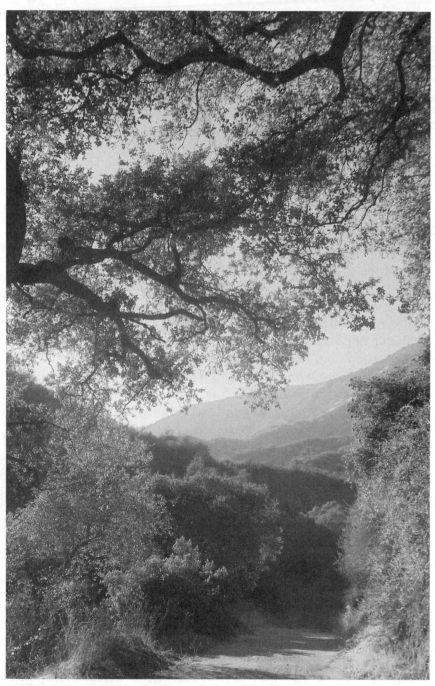

Marshall Canyon (Hike 91)

Introduction

"There is no exercise so beneficial, physically, mentally, or morally, nothing which gives so much of living for so little cost, as hiking our mountain and hill trails and sleeping under the stars."

So wrote the late Will Thrall—explorer, historian, author, and protector of the San Gabriel Mountains of Southern California.

Thrall's philosophy certainly applies today, in this age of high-pressure, rapid-paced urban life that engulfs so many Southern Californians. Fortunately, there are mountains practically in the backyard of Los Angeles that offer the harried city dweller a refreshing change of pace. Here, amid forest, chaparral, and stream, you can redeem and revitalize yourself in nature's unhurried environment. Traveling a wooded trail or scrambling along a rocky hillside, you can find solitude and gain perspective; you will come to discover the true value of wilderness to a civilization that too often places artificial values before real ones.

More than 135 years ago, in 1877, naturalist John Muir sampled the San Gabriels, found them wild and trailless, and described the range as "more rigidly inaccessible . . . than any other I ever attempted to penetrate." Great change has come to the San Gabriels since Muir's excursion. This once-primitive high country that he so vividly described in his classic *The Mountains of California* is today crisscrossed with paved highways, unpaved side roads, trails, and firebreaks. Yet wilderness is here for anyone who will leave behind pavement and campground to seek it on the numerous footpaths within range.

This guidebook represents a concerted effort to acquaint Southern Californians with the intimate parts of the San Gabriels—the regions away from highways and byways where nature remains relatively undisturbed. One hundred hiking trips take the reader and prospective hiker into almost every nook and cranny of the range. They vary from easy one-hour strolls to all-day and overnight rambles involving

1

many miles of walking and many elevation changes, from excursions to satisfy novice hikers to challenging ones for veteran adventurers. For history buffs, there are tours of the Mount Lowe Railway and the Echo Mountain ruins; for nature lovers, there are samplings of five wilderness areas, forever left to their natural states; for peak baggers, there are routes up almost all of the major summits of the range.

The San Gabriels are laced with trails and fire roads—some well maintained and easy to follow, others nearly forgotten due to erosion and overgrowth. The great majority of trips in this guidebook are on maintained trails and should offer no problems to the hiker. However, the writers have included a handful of cross-country excursions and trailless peak climbs in regions well worth visiting but not served by standard routes. For these trips, directions have been presented in greater detail.

The authors have rewalked, recorded, and researched all trips in this volume, most of them in recent years. Every effort has been made to present the information as accurately and as explicitly as possible. Nevertheless, the prospective hiker should be aware that several factors—some of them unique to the Southern California mountains—may make some of this information out of date in an amazingly short span of time. The first is the rapid growth of chaparral—the rigid, thorny brush that covers 80% of San Gabriel mountain slopes. A trail through this brushy maze, if not continually maintained, can become overgrown and virtually impassable in three years or fewer. Second is fire, the danger of which is extreme during late summer and fall, when the chaparral becomes tinder-dry. Fire denudes hillsides of vegetation, leaving them subject to dirt slippage and rockslides. Third is flood. Winter rainfall is generally moderate in the Southern California mountains (compared to the Sierra Nevada and other northern ranges), but every few years, deluges occur that are particularly destructive to canyon trails. On fire-ravaged hillsides, water erosion can be severe, obliterating large sections of trail. Last is the continual reworking, regrading, and rebuilding of maintained trails by the US Forest Service and volunteer conservation groups. Sometimes part of a trail is redirected along a different route, or road closures require different origination points. Such changes will probably affect only a few of the trips described herein, but if you are unfamiliar with the area in which you plan to hike, it is best to inquire at a ranger station before the trip.

To inquire about fire conditions, and for general questions concerning forest entry, contact the following US Forest Service facilities:

Monday–Friday:
Angeles National Forest headquarters 626-574-1613
Los Angeles River Ranger District 818-899-1900
San Gabriel River Ranger District 626-335-1251
Santa Clara/Mojave River Ranger District 661-269-2825

Saturday–Sunday:
Big Pines Information Center 760-249-3504
Mount Baldy Visitor Center 909-982-2829
Clear Creek Information Station 626-821-6764
Grassy Hollow Visitor Center 626-821-6737

This book is titled *Trails of the Angeles* because 95% of the San Gabriel Mountains are within Angeles National Forest. However, the eastern end of the range—from the great Baldy–Telegraph–Ontario Ridge to Cajon Pass—is in San Bernardino National Forest. This section boasts some of the finest high country in the mountains, and it has been included because it belongs here better than with the topographically different San Bernardino Mountains several miles east. (Refer to John W. Robinson's *San Bernardino Mountain Trails* for 100 trips in the latter range.)

The trips listed here are just a beginning. More than 100 hikes are possible in the San Gabriels, crisscrossed as these mountains are by walking routes. Furthermore, various combinations of routes described here are possible, particularly if you can arrange for car shuttles. You could spend a decade rambling through the range and still not have completely explored the mountains.

We hope that this guidebook will give you the knowledge that can make an outing in the San Gabriels an enjoyable and meaningful experience. Learn and heed forest regulations, follow route directions, become familiar with the area, have proper equipment, and use good sense. Never leave the trailhead without this preparation. The mountains are no place to travel alone, unbriefed, ill equipped, or in poor condition. Enter their portals with the enthusiasm of adventure tempered with respect, forethought, and common sense. The mountains belong to those who are wise as well as willing.

The San Gabriel Mountains

As long as humans have lived in the Los Angeles Basin, we have looked at the San Gabriel Mountains. Whether phantomlike behind a veil of brownish haze, sharply etched against a blue winter sky, or playing hide-and-seek with billowing clouds, they are a familiar scene on the northern skyline.

As mountains go, the San Gabriels are a gentle range. Ridgelines are sinuous rather than jagged, summits rounded rather than angular, and slopes tapered rather than sheer. Although they present a formidable barrier to north-south travel, their elevations and topographical features do not compare with the sky-piercing crags of the Sierra Nevada.

The San Gabriels form a great roof over the Southern California coastal lowlands, covering an area that reaches from seaward slopes across to the Mojave Desert and that extends west to east 68 miles from The Ridge Route to Cajon Pass. It can be said that the mountains act as both hero and villain to the Southland's millions: they protect the coastal plains from the desert's harshness and gather moisture from Pacific storms, but at the same time they increase urban air pollution by locking in air masses.

Geologists tell us that the range is a massive block of the Earth's crust, separated from the surrounding landscape by a network of major faults—the San Andreas Fault on the north, the San Gabriel and Sierra Madre Faults on the south, and the Soledad Fault on the west. The great block itself, in turn, is fractured by numerous subsidiary faults. The result is a surface that is extremely uneven. Eons of erosive stream action have cut deep V-shaped canyons, further accentuating the unevenness. The surface rocks are fractured and intermixed in great confusion, forming a heterogeneous mixture of crystalline limestone, schists, and quartzites, which have been invaded by intrusive granites and other igneous rocks, all forming a most complicated mass.

Covering about 80% of this wrinkled mountain mass is a thick blanket of stiff, thorny shrubs and dwarf trees collectively called chaparral: chamise, scrub oak, yucca, wild lilac, mountain mahogany, laurel, snowbrush (whitethorn), chinquapin, and that unpopular champion of all rigidity, manzanita. This elfin forest, where it has not recently been burned off—for it grows quickly back—fastens securely to hillsides, seizing every square foot not preempted by timber or crag. It swarms over hot, exposed slopes whose conditions it alone can endure, spreading until it forms an almost impenetrable collar between the foothills and the high pine country.

Chaparral has been damned as too low to give shade, too high to see over, and too thick to go through. Anyone so foolish as to venture off road or trail and crawl through this brushy maze will soon come to believe that there is a personal hostility in the unyielding branches and scratchy leaves.

A different experience awaits those who consider this elfin forest as a friend to visit, not as an enemy to thrash through. In bloom, much of the chaparral is sprinkled with colorful flowers. And what is more pleasing to the nature lover than ceanothus blooming into misty blue or white, California laurel unfolding masses of yellow flowers, or wild lilac giving forth its sweet aroma after a spring rain? Chaparral is also valuable as a soil cover; where it has been burned off, rain rushes down the hillsides, causing severe erosion on the slopes and flooding in the canyons.

Below the chaparral belt, in the canyons, a luxuriant cover of sycamore, live oak, alder, and bay trees shields sparkling streams from the sun's glare. Above the chaparral, and sometimes as enclaves within it, is a cool, stately world of conifers: first big-cone Douglas-firs, and then—progressively higher—Jeffrey and ponderosa pines, Coulter pines, incense cedars, sugar pines, white firs, and lodgepole pines. On the highest ridges, subalpine conditions reign, and gnarled limber pines live a marginal existence among windswept crags.

The wildlife of the San Gabriel Mountains is timid—as well it should be. Humans have preempted most of the range, crowding out animals that once roamed in abundance. Some species are gone completely: no longer does the giant California condor soar overhead (although the occasional straggler sometimes wanders over from Ventura County), nor the mammoth grizzly bear prowl the forest. Both disappeared from here shortly after the turn of the 20th century. Often seen in the San

Gabriels and in nearby foothill communities is the black bear; natural-
ists estimate their number to be anywhere from 250 to 300 and they
seem to be on the increase. In the remote recesses of the range, an estimated 250 Nelson bighorn sheep scratch out a living, and the population has suffered a steep decline in the past few decades; experts are
unsure of the exact causes. You must walk far from the highway to see
these noble animals, deep into the rugged San Gabriel and Cucamonga
Wildernesses or high up on the stony battlements of Iron Mountain.

The most abundant large mammal in the San Gabriels is the
California mule deer, usually yellow-brown in summer, gray in winter, its many-pronged antlers growing to considerable size. Preying
on the deer are a growing number of mountain lions, perhaps 40 or
50 in the whole range. In recent years, sightings of these agile beasts
have increased, and several well-publicized attacks have occurred.
Although the odds of an encounter are slight, hikers should be vigi-
lant, and children should never be left unattended. Smaller mammals
include the bobcat, ring-tailed cat, gray fox, weasel, skunk, and a host
of squirrels and chipmunks. The region's most common creature considered sometimes dangerous to humans is the western rattlesnake,
abundant below 6,000 feet, and sometimes seen up to 8,000 feet.
However, most rattlers are not very aggressive and will move away
when approached.

Geographically, the San Gabriels are for most of their length made
up of two roughly parallel ranges. The northern, inland range is the
longer and loftier, extending from Mount Gleason and Mount Pacifico
eastward past the 8,000-foot and 9,000-foot summits of Waterman,
Williamson, Islip, Hawkins, Throop, and Baden-Powell, and climax-
ing near its eastern end in the only summit over 10,000 feet—Mount
San Antonio (Old Baldy) and its cluster of satellite peaks. The southern, or front, range, though neither as long nor as high, is equally as
rugged. Two of its summits—Strawberry and San Gabriel—exceed
6,000 feet, and 10 others exceed 5,000 feet. Below the peaks is a complex of deep, shaded canyons, extending well up into the higher parts
of the range. The range's major watershed is the San Gabriel River,
whose three main forks and countless tributaries drain fully 20% of
the mountain precipitation. Other important watersheds are Pacoima,
Little Tujunga, Big Tujunga, Arroyo Seco, Santa Anita, San Antonio,
and Lytle Creek Canyons on the south slope of the range, and Little
Rock and Big Rock Creeks on the north.

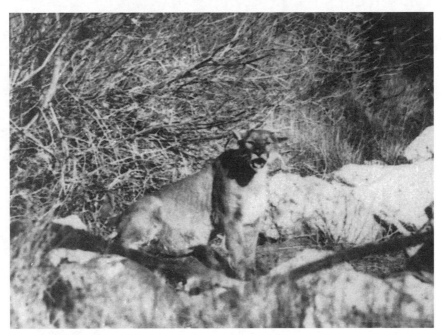

Mountain lion near Chilao

Finally, there is the Liebre Mountain–Sawmill Mountain–Sierra Pelona country to the northwest of the San Gabriels proper, beyond the great wind gap of Soledad Canyon. Geographers disagree on whether this gentle mountain region of long whale-backed ridges and shallow canyons belongs to the San Gabriels, the Tehachapis, or to neither. But it is part of Angeles National Forest and it is good hiking country, so it is included here.

Other mountain ranges in California are higher, more jagged, more bedecked with ice and snow, more breathtaking, or more primitive. But no other is so accessible to so many people for so little effort—and year-round. When winter's white mantle closes off the high country, the woodsy canyons and green-velvet foothills become refreshing, delightful, and inviting. And then, in turn, when summer's swelter-ing dryness invades canyon and foothill, the high mountains once again beckon. For this all-season aspect, and for the San Gabriels themselves—ageless, rock-ribbed, and aromatic with the restoring scents of forest and chaparral—shall we ever be thankful.

Humans in the San Gabriels

Humans have entered the San Gabriels in almost every conceivable manner. We have come into the mountains for a multitude of reasons. And we have come in great numbers. Few mountain ranges anywhere have been so viewed, swarmed over, dug into, and built upon by the human species.

What draws us to the mountains? Is it curiosity? The promise of adventure? The excitement of hunting and fishing? The chance of a better livelihood? The quest for mineral wealth? The longing to redeem and revitalize oneself, away from the hustle of urban life? The need for something spiritual or ego-satisfying? The long pageant of humans in the San Gabriels reveals all these motives, along with some that are not so readily identified. The fascination of the canyons, the ridges, the peaks, and the little flats that lie deep in the mountains has attracted human visitors since humans first made their home in Southern California. People have come to the mountains, have seen, have lingered, and in many cases have remained for life.

One might suppose that the San Gabriels would be worn out (ecologically) by all this human activity. Some parts are, particularly in the front range. Fortunately, though, there are other areas where human impact has been minimal, where nature still rules—thanks to the protective efforts of a handful of people who, for a variety of reasons ranging from enlightened self-interest to aesthetic values, have fought to save the mountains and the forests for the benefit of all. Humankind is not totally shortsighted, although we often appear to be.

The first humans in the San Gabriels were American Indian peoples of Shoshonean stock—Gabrielinos in the southern foothills, Fernandeños in the western canyons, and Serranos in the eastern and northern high country. (These tribal names were assigned by anthropologists. The groups named Gabrielinos and Fernandeños were associated with Missions San Gabriel and San Fernando, respectively. However, the indigenous name Tongva is preferred by American Indian activists and Gabrielino descendants. Serrano is derived from the Spanish word meaning "mountaineer.") Other tribal groups in the Liebre–Sawmill–Sierra Pelona country were the Alliklik and the Kitanemuk peoples, also Shoshonean. Though their homes were generally below the mountains, these peoples depended heavily on the San Gabriel range. The mountains supplied them with food, water, and materials for building and hunting. For food, they hunted deer and rabbits and gathered acorns and pine nuts. They took water from the streams that gushed down from great heights. Chaparral was an abundant source of many necessities. Manzanita berries were pressed for cider, and the leaves were smoked. Greasewood provided arrow shafts for hunting. Yucca fibers were used to make nets and ropes.

To obtain these materials, and to visit and trade with other peoples across the range, American Indians made the first footpaths into the mountains. According to Will Thrall, foremost collector of San Gabriel Mountains history, who personally searched out these ancient routes at a time when they could still be followed, the main Shoshone trail across the range ascended Millard Canyon, traversed behind Mount Lowe to Red Box Saddle, descended the West Fork of the San Gabriel River to Valley Forge Canyon, climbed up that canyon to Barley Flats, went down and across the head of Big Tujunga Canyon and up to Pine (Charlton) Flat, and continued on to the west end of Chilao. Here, the trail forked. One branch followed the high country northeast to Buckhorn, and then went down the South Fork of Little Rock Creek to the desert. The other branch dropped northwest into upper Alder Creek, and then ascended Indian Ridge (where traces of the old footpath can still be seen) to Sheep Camp Spring on the west slope of Mount Pacifico, and dropped down Santiago Canyon to Little Rock Creek and along it to the desert. Another cross-range trail ascended the North Fork of the San Gabriel River, climbed over Windy Gap, and descended the South Fork of Big Rock Creek to the desert. For perhaps two or three centuries before the arrival of the white settlers, these and many shorter canyon trails were trod by hundreds of American Indians every year.

The arrival of the Spaniards changed life in the pleasant valleys below the mountains forever. In 1771, along the grassy banks of the Rio Hondo, Mission San Gabriel Arcángel was founded, and soon thereafter, the Gabrielinos were incorporated into the mission community. Mission San Fernando Rey de España, founded in 1797, became the home of the less-numerous Fernandeños. At the height of mission activity—around 1800—these two outposts of the cross numbered some 2,000 American Indians in their widespread flocks.

Several decades later came the era of the great ranchos, bringing a pastoral way of life to the valleys. These spacious cattle ranches that spread out below the south slopes of the range bore the familiar names of San Fernando, Tujunga, La Cañada, San Pascual, Santa Anita, Azusa de Duarte, and San Jose.

The Spanish and Mexican Californios used the mountains very little except as a source of water. When there were buildings to be constructed, woodcutters sometimes took timber from the lower canyons. Vaqueros did some hunting in the canyons and foothills. Grizzly bears, numerous in the range then, were stalked and captured, and then dragged to the bull ring in the Pueblo of Los Angeles to be sacrificed in brutal bear-bull contests.

There is no evidence that the Spaniards ever penetrated into the heart of the mountains, although they certainly explored the fringes. Gaspar de Portolá and Pedro Fages, on their epic journey northward in 1769, toiled through the narrow canyon of San Fernando Pass and found "high, barren hills, very difficult for beasts of burden" before dropping into pleasant Newhall Valley. On another path-finding trip in 1772, Fages crossed the eastern end of the range in the vicinity of Cajon Pass and continued northwest below the northern ramparts of the mountains, discovering the Joshua trees. Fray Francisco Garcés, the missionary-explorer-martyr, explored both sides of the range in 1776. Fray José María Zalvidea almost circled what is now Angeles National Forest in 1806.

It was the Spaniards who gave the mountains their name—two names, in fact, that have existed side by side until relatively recent years. In 1776 Garcés referred to the range as Sierra de San Gabriel, borrowing the name of the nearby mission, and this name was used in Spanish records frequently in ensuing years. But the mission padres usually referred to the range as Sierra Madre ("mother range"). Both San Gabriel and Sierra Madre were in common usage until 1927, when the U.S. Board on Geographic Names finally ruled in favor of the former. Today San Gabriel Mountains is almost universally accepted.

With the coming of the Anglos—from the 1840s onward—the San Gabriels began to receive more attention. Prospectors, hunters, bandits, homesteaders, and squatters were pioneers in unveiling the secrets of the mountains. These hardy individuals first entered the wooded canyons, and then forged their way over the ridges and into the hidden heart of the range—terrain the rancheros had scorned.

Stories of gold in the San Gabriels go back as far as the 1770s, but not until 1842, when Francisco Lopez discovered gold clinging to the roots of a cluster of wild onions in Placerita Canyon, near present-day Newhall, was there what might be called a gold rush. The San Fernando Placers, as the discovery was called, were worked on and off for about a decade, until strikes elsewhere drew the miners away. By far, the largest gold strike in the San Gabriels occurred on the East Fork of the San Gabriel River. The precious metal was discovered in the canyon gravels in 1854, and for the next seven years the East Fork was the scene of frenzied activity, an estimated $2 million in gold being recovered. A smaller strike occurred in Big Santa Anita Canyon about the same time. During the next half century, prospectors rushed into the mountains at every rumor of bonanza, tearing up hillsides in their frantic search for wealth.

Bandits, including Jack Powers, Salomon Pico, Juan Flores, and the legendary Tiburcio Vásquez, turned to the San Gabriels for refuge. They drove stolen cattle and horses up the canyons and pastured them in backcountry flats. Utilizing the faint network of old American Indian trails, these outlaws established isolated hideouts deep in the mountains.

The pioneer trail builder in the San Gabriels was Benjamin Wilson, who in 1864 reworked an old American Indian path up Little Santa Anita Canyon to the top of the mountain that now bears his name. During the next three decades, trails were blazed up all the major canyons of the front range, some of them continuing over the ridges and into the backcountry. In increasing numbers, homesteaders and squatters followed these trails and found favorite spots on which to build their cabins. The names of many of these early mountain men have endured to the present, attached to canyons, camps, and peaks—Wilson, Millard, Henninger, Newcomb, Chantry, Chilao, Islip, and Dawson, to name a few.

Almost all these pioneers came into the mountains for utilitarian reasons—to mine gold, to cut timber, to find refuge, to pasture livestock, or to establish a home. Around 1885 a new reason for going to the mountains arose—recreation. Great numbers of San Gabriel Valley residents journeyed to Mount Wilson on weekends and holidays to enjoy the cool mountain air and take in the fabulous panorama. (This was before air pollution muddled Southland skies.) Hunters entered the range seeking big game, plentiful in the San Gabriels until around the turn of the century. Grizzly bears, black bears, deer, mountain sheep, and mountain lions were stalked by bands of thrill-seeking hunters who penetrated far into the mountains. Sportsmen packed in for a week's fishing on the trout-filled West Fork of the San Gabriel River. For the less energetic, there were Sunday afternoon picnics in such woodsy haunts as Millard and Eaton Canyons.

Other people entered the mountains for a different reason—exploitation. Most Americans of that day assumed that our natural resources were inexhaustible and therefore there was no need to conserve them. Lumber was needed to fuel Southern California's great boom of the 1880s; why not use the timber close at hand? Indiscriminate cutting of forest trees appeared imminent. Furthermore, the value of chaparral for the mountain watershed was little understood. Brush fires, some deliberately set by cattlemen to clear land for grazing, raged across the mountains until extinguished by rain. Fortunately, some farsighted residents in Los Angeles and the San Gabriel Valley became alarmed at this exploitation and devastation of the local mountains, and they began working to preserve the lands.

One of these was Abbot Kinney, a rancher, botanist, and land developer who lived at his Kinneloa Ranch above Altadena. Kinney is best remembered as the creator of Venice, the Southern California beach town that once had canals for streets, but it was as chairman of California's first Board of Forestry that he did his most important work. In the first report of the Board of Forestry to Governor George Stoneman in 1886, Kinney urged "intelligent supervision of the forest land and brush lands of California, with a view to their preservation." This California movement for forest conservation, sparked by Kinney and others, soon became part of a national movement. John Muir, using his eloquence in a series of magazine articles urging forest protection, was the leading spokesman.

Congress finally responded by passing the Forest Reserve Act of 1891, granting the president the authority "to set apart and reserve

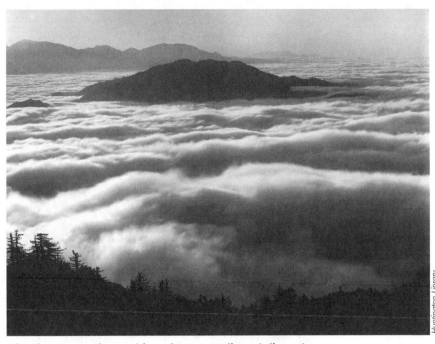

Huntington Library

Clouds over southeast ridge of Mount Wilson (Hike 45)

. . . any part of the public lands wholly or in part covered with timber or undergrowth." As a result of this act, and strong pressure from Southern California civic leaders, President Benjamin Harrison signed the bill establishing the San Gabriel Timberland Reserve on December 20, 1892. This was the first forest reserve in California and the second in the United States. (The first was the Yellowstone Park Timberland Reserve in Wyoming, established by presidential proclamation on September 16, 1891.) The designation was at first rather ineffectual; for one thing, forest rangers were not assigned until 1898. But gradually the San Gabriel Timberland Reserve was brought under efficient forest management and protection. In 1907 the name was changed to San Gabriel National Forest, and the following year it became what we know today—Angeles National Forest. A succession of capable supervisors—Everett Thomas, Theodore Lukens, Rush Charlton, William Mendenhall, Sim Jarvi, William Dresser, and Paul Sweetland—have made the Angeles one of the most effectively run national forests in the nation.

Worldwide fame came to the San Gabriels in the 1890s with construction of the Mount Lowe Railway, considered one of the

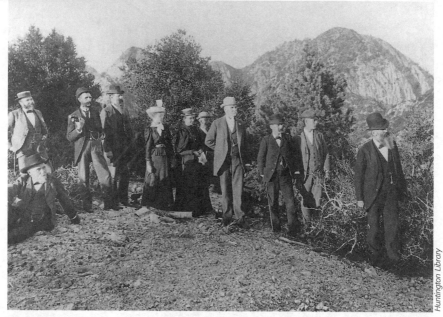

Huntington Library

Professor Thaddeus S. C. Lowe (center) and party on Mount Lowe (1892)

engineering wonders of its time. This breathtaking cable incline and trolley ride—along with associated hotels in Rubio Canyon, atop Echo Mountain, and on the slopes of Mount Lowe—was the brainchild of inventor Thaddeus S. C. Lowe and engineer David Macpherson. The famed mountain railway-resort complex attracted more than 3 million visitors during its 43 years of operation.

The human quest for scientific knowledge played its part in the story of the mountains too. In the days before city lights and air pollution interfered with sky viewing, Mount Wilson's broad summit was ideal for astronomical observation. The first telescope on Mount Wilson was the 13-incher of Harvard University Observatory, placed on the summit in 1889 (but removed the following year). The year 1904 saw the beginning of the Carnegie Institute's famed Mount Wilson Observatory, one of the 20th century's great scientific ventures. Largely through the initiative and enthusiasm of astronomer George Ellery Hale, several of the world's greatest telescopes were erected on the mountaintop, the most important being the 60-inch reflector (1908), the 150-foot solar tower telescope (1912), and the

100-inch Hooker reflector (1917), the latter the world's largest optical telescope for 31 years.

Before highways crisscrossed the San Gabriels, the mountains were the delight of hikers. Mountain historians call the period from about 1895 to 1938 the Great Hiking Era. Multitudes of lowland residents enjoyed their weekends and holidays rambling over the range. Trails that today are almost deserted vibrated to the busy tramp of boots and the merry singing of hikers. The mountains were a local frontier for exploration and a challenge to the hardy. For some, hiking was simply a favorite sport; for others, it was almost a religion. Trail resorts sprang up to offer hospitality, food, and lodging to hikers. Such places as Switzer's, Opid's, Colby's, Loomis's, Sturtevant's, and Roberts's were visited by thousands every season.

A strange combination of disasters and "progress" brought the Great Hiking Era to a close. The disasters were a series of fires and consequent floods, the great destructive torrent of March 1938 being the final blow. Overnight, miles of canyon trails were obliterated. "Progress" took the form of the Angeles Crest Highway, begun in 1929. Relentlessly, the great asphalt thoroughfare snaked its way into the heart of the mountains, reaching Red Box in 1934, Charlton Flat in 1937, and Chilao a year later. By 1941 it had inched its way across Cloudburst Summit and reached that most isolated of backcountry haunts, Buckhorn. Places that once required a day or two of strenuous hiking were now accessible in an hour of driving. One by one, the old trail resorts succumbed. As one old-timer sadly reflected, "Only people who hike for the love of hiking use these trails now." The Angeles Crest Highway, more than anything else, changed the pattern of our use of the San Gabriels.

In recent years, great numbers of people have visited the San Gabriels, the vast majority by automobile, and visitation is increasing. Each year there are an estimated 3.5 million visits to the Angeles National Forest, making the Angeles one of the most heavily used national forests in the United States.

As the use has increased, the wilderness aspect of the mountains has been nearly destroyed. Other than the specially set-aside wilderness areas and a few other small, isolated regions, the San Gabriels have in recent years become not much more than a king-size backyard playground for Los Angeles County. Some say that this is as it should be, but recent ecological studies have tended to show that wilderness undisturbed by humans plays a vital part in nature's delicate balance among living things. What happens when there is no wilderness left? Southern California appears headed in that direction.

Angeles National Forest today encompasses 694,187 acres. Within this mountain area are 1,030 miles of roads, 697 miles of riding and hiking trails, 66 public campgrounds, 36 picnic areas, 505 summer residences, five wilderness areas, and three winter sports areas.

The future of the San Gabriels—as well as all other mountain ranges—rests with the population that lives nearby. In the words of mountain historian Charles Clark Vernon, "They are truly a gift to the people." What the people will do with this gift of nature remains to be seen.

The Station Fire

What became the largest fire in the history of the San Gabriels—and the largest in Los Angeles County history—began inauspiciously enough on August 26, 2009, near the Angeles Crest Highway just above La Cañada. With several other large fires burning around the state, it received little notice at first and was nearly extinguished that first evening. However, overnight the fire gained strength, and by the next day it was out of control and began to spread, ultimately consum-

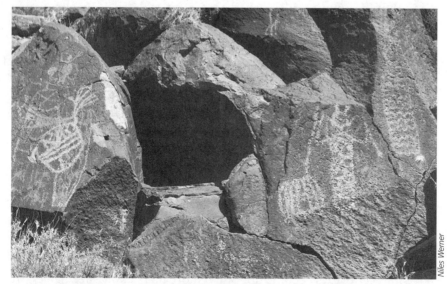

American Indian petroglyphs near Big Pine

ing more than 160,000 acres, approximately one-fourth of the Angeles National Forest. It was later determined that the fire was started by a still-unknown arsonist. Two Los Angeles County firefighters lost their lives battling the blaze when their truck tumbled off a roadway in the Mount Gleason area.

In the aftermath of the fire—finally extinguished in mid-October—a large swath of the forest was officially closed to all entry. It has slowly reopened in stages, but as of this writing—spring 2013—portions of the Arroyo Seco and upper Big Tujunga areas are still classified as off-limits to hikers. The recently opened areas will still take years to recover fully. And the pine-and-fir

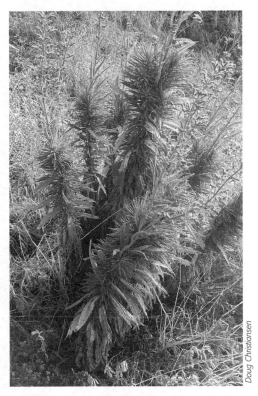

Watch out for poodle-dog bush!

forests that once clothed the higher mountaintops and flats—such as Mount Gleason, Charlton Flats, and Barley Flats—may never regain their former beauty.

The authors have done their best to hike the trails in the burn area and note any changes; however, it is advisable to check ahead with the US Forest Service to verify current conditions before venturing into any recently opened areas.

Turricula, also known as poodle-dog bush, is a fire-following plant that has become widespread in Station Fire burn areas. It is a woody shrub with stems branching out from the base up to 6 feet in length, and it sports purple flowers that bloom during summer. Hikers should give this toxic plant a wide berth, as any contact can result in serious skin irritation much worse than that resulting from poison oak.

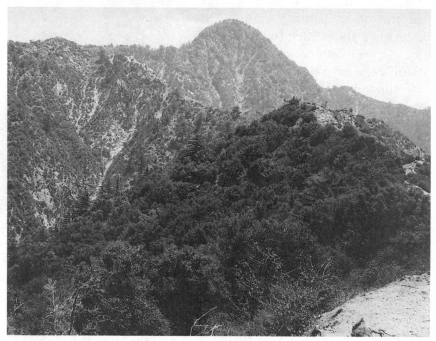

Strawberry Peak (Hike 38)

Hiking Hints

Traveling a mountain trail, away from centers of civilization, is a unique experience in Southern California living. It brings intimate association with nature—communion with the earth, the forest, the chaparral, the wildlife, and the clear sky. A great responsibility accompanies this experience—the obligation to keep the mountains as you found them. Being considerate of the wilderness rights of others will make the mountain adventures of those who follow equally rewarding.

As a mountain visitor, you should become familiar with the rules of wilderness courtesy outlined below.

Trails

Never cut switchbacks. This practice breaks down trails and hastens erosion. Take care not to dislodge rocks that might fall on hikers below you. Improve and preserve trails, as by clearing away loose rocks (carefully) and removing branches. Report any trail damage and broken or misplaced signs to a ranger.

Off Trail

Restrain the impulse to blaze trees or to build cairns where not essential. Let the next fellow find his way as you did.

Mountain Bikes

Mountain bikers need to respect the rights and the safety of hikers and horseback riders and should follow sound conservation practices. Yield right-of-way to other trail users. Control your speed. Stay off muddy trails, and do not shortcut switchbacks. Mountain biking is permissible on most forest trails but is prohibited in wilderness areas and on the Pacific Crest Trail.

Campgrounds

Spread your gear in an already-cleared area, and build your fire in a campground stove. Don't disarrange the camp by making hard-to-eradicate ramparts of rock for fireplaces or windbreaks. Rig tents and tarps with line tied to rocks or trees; never put nails in trees. For your campfire, use fallen wood only; do not cut standing trees or break off branches. Use the campground latrine. Place litter in the litter can or carry it out. Leave the campground cleaner than you found it.

Fire

Fire is the greatest danger in the Southern California mountains; act accordingly. Smoking is permitted only in campgrounds, places of habitation, and vehicles. Report a mountain fire immediately to the US Forest Service.

Litter

Along the trail, place candy wrappers, raisin boxes, orange peels, and so on in your pocket or pack for later disposal; throw nothing on the trail. Pick up litter you find along the trail or in camp. More than almost anything else, litter detracts from the wilderness scene. Remember, you can take it with you.

Noise

Boisterous conduct is out of harmony in a wilderness experience. Be a considerate hiker and camper. Don't ruin another's enjoyment of the mountains.

Hiker Ethics

Human life and well-being take precedence over most everything else—in the mountains as elsewhere. If a hiker or camper is in trouble, help in any way you can. Give comfort or first aid, and then hurry to a ranger station for help.

Maps

It is important to know where you are in relation to roads, camp-grounds, landmarks, and so on, and to have a general understanding of the lay of the land. For this orientation there is no substitute for a good map. Unless your trip is very short, and over a well-marked route, you should carry a map.

Besides the shaded relief trail map that accompanies this book, there are two other types of maps that will give you the picture you need of the San Gabriel Mountains. Each type has its advantages and disadvantages.

1. The US Forest Service sells recreation maps of each national forest. For the San Gabriels, you will need the maps of Angeles and San Bernardino National Forests. These maps show the highways, dirt roads, maintained trails, campgrounds, and major landmarks of the range, but not the topography. Their main advantages are that they give you an overall picture of the mountains and are fairly up-to-date, being revised frequently. Because they don't show topographic features or ground cover, they are virtually useless for cross-country travel. These maps can be obtained at most ranger stations in the two national forests. Or write to the forest headquarters:

Angeles National Forest
701 N. Santa Anita
Arcadia, CA 91006
626-574-1613

San Bernardino National Forest
602 South Tippecano Ave.
San Bernardino, CA 92408
909-382-2600

2. If you do much hiking, particularly cross-country, you will want
to use topographic ("topo") maps because they afford accurate information about the topography and the forest or brush cover. Topo
maps are available in several sizes and scales, but the best for the San
Gabriels, because they are the most up-to-date and show the greatest detail, are the U.S. Geological Survey's 7.5-minute topographic
quadrangle series. Their scale is approximately 2.5 inches to a mile;
the contour interval (elevation difference between contour lines) is
40 feet, and the area covered by each map is about 7 miles by 9 miles.
They show most maintained and many unmaintained trails, as well
as elevations, relief, watercourses, forest and brush cover, and man-
made structures. Learning to read these maps takes some practice, but
the savings in shoe leather and frayed temper make it a worthwhile
undertaking. Twenty-seven topo maps (in the 7.5-minute series)
cover the San Gabriel Mountains. The appropriate topo map(s) for
each trip is cited in the individual trip headings. Topo maps can be
bought at many sporting goods and mountaineering-ski shops, or can
be ordered online from the USGS website: **store.usgs.gov.**

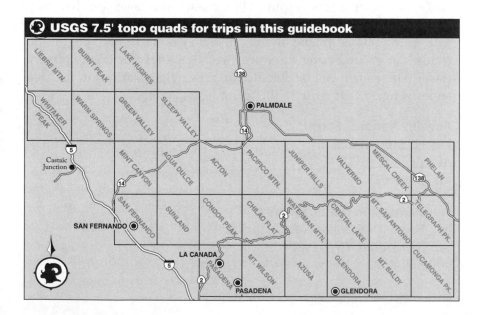

Using This Book

The hiking trips in this guide are arranged by geographical area, generally west to east. Information about each trip is divided into three parts: *Trip*, *Features*, and *Description*.

The **Trip** section gives vital statistics: where the hike starts and ends; the walking mileage and elevation gain or loss; a rating of easy, moderate, or strenuous; the best time of year to make the trip; and the appropriate U.S. Geological Survey topographic map or maps.

The **Features** section tells something of what you will see on the trip and gives information on the natural and human history of the area. It also contains suggestions for the particular trip, such as "wear lug-soled boots," or "bring fishing rod."

The **Description** section details driving and hiking routes. The driving directions are kept to the necessary minimum, while the walking route is described in detail. Also, hiking options that a trip presents are described.

The hikes have been graded as easy, moderate, or strenuous. An easy trip is usually 4 miles or less in horizontal distance, with less than a 500-foot elevation gain—suitable for beginners and children. A moderate trip—including the majority here—is a 5- to 10-mile hike, usually with less than a 2,500-foot elevation difference. You should be in fair physical condition for these, and children under age 12 might find the going difficult. Strenuous trips are all-day rambles involving many miles of hiking and much elevation gain and loss; they are only for those in top physical condition and with hiking experience. The most important criteria for grading a trip were mileage covered, elevation gain and loss, and condition of the trail. Of less significance were accessibility of terrain, availability of water, exposure to sun, and ground cover. Obviously, some of the latter criteria depend on the weather and the time of year: a 3-mile hike over open chaparral slopes can be miserable under the hot August sun but delightful in January's cool breeze and cloudiness.

A season recommendation is also included for each trip. This classification is particularly important in the lower, south-facing parts of the range, where fire danger in summer and fall often reaches what the US Forest Service calls Stage One. During Stage One, campfires are permitted only in stoves in designated campgrounds and picnic areas. Gas-type portable stoves may be used if you obtain a California campfire permit—available at any ranger station or visitor center. In conditions of extreme fire danger, the forest may be closed to entry off of major highways. In recent years a series of disastrous infernos has taken a heavy toll, both in property damage and in the cost required to fight the fires. The result is that wholesale closure of the forest during certain times, particularly the fall months, will increasingly be a common occurrence.

Wilderness Permits

There are five wilderness areas in the San Gabriels—Cucamonga, Sheep Mountain, San Gabriel, and, newly created in 2009, the Pleasant View Ridge and Magic Mountain Wilderness areas. A free permit is required for all entry into the Cucamonga Wilderness, and for entry into the Sheep Mountain Wilderness from the East Fork trailhead only.

National Forest Adventure Pass Requirement

A National Forest Adventure Pass is required to park your vehicle in any of the four national forests in Southern California. Adventure passes cost $30 for an annual pass or $5 for a day pass; they can be purchased at ranger stations, visitor centers, and many business establishments in or near the mountains. Be sure to display the pass prominently on your parked car—otherwise it will likely be ticketed and fined. **Please note that most of the trips covered in this book require you to display an Adventure Pass in your parked vehicle.** The following are the trips where you park on city streets, or that begin in a park with separate entrance fees, and do *not* require the pass: 5, 14–15, 23–28, 34, 39–40, 48–50, 67–68, and 91.

100 Hikes in the San Gabriels

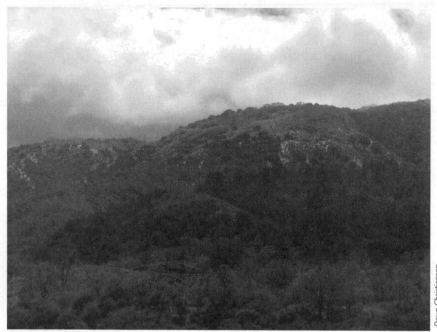

Liebre Mountain

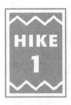

COUNTY ROAD N2 VIA HORSE TRAIL
TO LIEBRE MOUNTAIN

HIKE LENGTH: 6 miles round-trip; 1,700' elevation gain
DIFFICULTY: Moderate
SEASON: All year
TOPO MAP: *Liebre Mountain*

Features

The long whaleback of Liebre Mountain sprawls at the northwest corner of Angeles National Forest, where the Coast Ranges, the Tehachapis, and the San Gabriels all meld together in a wrinkled jumble. From Liebre's broad summit, you look north across golden-brown Antelope Valley to the Tehachapis, curving from west to northeast in a great arc; and if the day is clear, the southern ramparts of the Sierra Nevada are visible on the distant skyline. Southward, you peer into the gentle ridge-and-canyon country of the Cienaga and Fish Canyon watersheds.

This is delightful mountain country, especially in spring, when snow patches linger on north slopes, the California black oak is clothing itself with reddish leaves, and aromatic white sage is blooming in the foothills. This is the home of the gray pine, a hardy dweller on semiarid slopes, easily identifiable by its gray-green needles, large cones (second in size only to the Coulter pine), and multiforked trunk. Also on the mountainside are big-cone Douglas-firs and some rather large scrub oaks. Occasional junipers and piñon pines bear testimony to the blending of mountain and desert here.

This trip follows the historic old Horse Trail, now part of the Pacific Crest Trail but once used to drive horses from the Tejon Ranch to Los Angeles, steeply up the forested north slope of Liebre Mountain from Horse Trail Flat to the summit. Do it in leisurely fashion to fully appreciate the desert view and the unique combination of forest trees and chaparral. It's a long drive from Los Angeles, but the mountainside is remote, peaceful, and beautiful—well worth the effort.

Description

From I-5, 4 miles south of Gorman, turn east onto CA 138. After 4.5 miles, turn right (southeast) onto the Old Ridge Route. Follow the latter 2.5 miles, and then turn left (east) onto County Road N2. Drive this road 4.2 miles, to a high point just before the road begins to descend. Turn right (south) and drive on dirt tracks about 100 feet to the oak-shaded parking area. Be sure to display your Adventure Pass on your vehicle's dashboard.

At the upper edge of the parking area is the Pacific Crest Trail, the southbound section climbing west, the northbound dropping southeast. Take the southbound PCT, which ascends the mountainside. (If you start descending, you're on the wrong trail segment.) You switchback up through live oaks and gray pines, with far-ranging views over Antelope Valley to the Tehachapis. After 2 miles you pass Wilderness Camp to your right. A table and fire ring are here, but there's no water. (Water can usually be found in Horse Camp Canyon just behind and steeply down from the camp; the easiest way to get water is to continue up the trail 0.25 mile, where the descent into the canyon is less steep.) You continue switchbacking upward, under a cool canopy of pines and oaks. Near the top your trail becomes an old jeep track. About 60 yards before you reach the crest and a junction with Forest Road 7N23, turn right and scramble to the small rock cairn that marks the 5,791-foot summit of Liebre Mountain.

Return the way you came. Or, with a car shuttle, meet your transportation on FR 7N23 on the crest of the long Liebre hogback. To drive to the crest, follow the Old Ridge Route to its crossing of the west end of Liebre Mountain, 5 miles up from CA 138, and then turn left (east) onto FR 7N23. Follow the latter, a narrow dirt road, steep in places, to the crest.

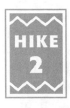

SAWMILL MOUNTAIN RIDGE TO ATMORE MEADOWS, GILLETTE MINE, BEAR CANYON

HIKE LENGTH: 14 miles round-trip;
1,700' elevation gain and loss
DIFFICULTY: Strenuous
SEASON: All year
TOPO MAPS: *Burnt Peak, Liebre Mountain*

Features

Just south of the great whalebacks of Liebre and Sawmill Mountains lies some of the loneliest mountain country in Angeles National Forest. This is a region of long, meandering canyons, gentle ridges, and rounded summits. Chaparral is king here; its prickly greenness blankets everything except the canyon bottoms, where tall oaks and sycamores grow and there are a few isolated stands of big-cone Douglas-firs and pines. This is also the realm of California mule deer, a favorite of hunters. Hikers are rare, yet the country has a multitude of trails. Unfortunately, many of the trails are presently overgrown, no longer maintained by the US Forest Service. You must be prepared for some bushwhacking, and a few spots of trail are so overgrown that it is difficult to follow. This trip is not recommended for beginners.

This trip begins near Atmore Meadows, contours over slopes of scrub oaks, manzanitas, yuccas, chamises, and chamises' cousin red shanks, and then drops into Bear Canyon. (There are three Bear Canyons in the Angeles.) Here, you visit the ruins of the Gillette Mine, a gold-and-silver prospect dating from the 1880s. En route you pass several trail junctions, each offering opportunities for further discovery (*see* Description below). The best time of year is spring, when there is still water in the canyons, when oaks and sycamores are dressing themselves in red and green, and when the air is sweet with the perfume of wet chaparral. Autumn is crisp and dry, yet the leaves of the black oaks on Sawmill Mountain—some yellow, some almost bright red—produce a vivid splash of color against the drab background.

Description

From I-5, 4 miles south of Gorman, turn right (east) onto CA 138. After 4.5 miles turn right again (southeast) onto the Old Ridge Route. About 2.5 miles farther, turn left (east) onto County Road N2. Follow CR N2 13 miles to Bushnell Summit, where it intersects

Forest Road 7N23 leading right (southwest) up Sawmill Mountain.
Follow CR 7N23 for 3 miles to the crest of the mountain, and then
turn right (west) along the ridgetop. Continue 3.5 miles to the intersection with the Atmore Meadows spur road, CR 7N19. Park here.
Be sure to display your Adventure Pass on your parked vehicle.

Walk around the locked gate and follow CR 7N19 down to a
horseshoe bend just short of the abandoned Atmore Meadows
Campground, 2 miles.

The trail leads south from this horseshoe bend in the road, passes
a seepage, and in 0.5 mile reaches a junction. The left fork descends
into Fish Canyon (*see* Hike 3). Go right, across chaparral slopes to a
prominent saddle. Here, the mostly overgrown trail contours along
the side of the ridge and climbs slightly before descending into Bear
Canyon, 4 miles from CR 7N19. It's easy to miss a switchback here,
thanks to overgrown chaparral, so proceed carefully.

In Bear Canyon you meet a dirt road coming over the ridge from
Knapp Ranch. Go left and follow the road down-canyon 0.5 mile
to the Gillette Mine remains, marked by tailings and rusted metal.
Across the creek is a more recent mine owned by the Benco Mining
Company, not being developed as of this writing.

Return the same way, almost all uphill. You have the option of
continuing 3 miles down Bear Canyon to its merger with Cienaga
Canyon. However, the old trail has largely disappeared and you must
follow the creek and negotiate some brushy areas. Unfortunately,
the once-scenic trail over Redrock Mountain ridge and down to Fish
Canyon (*see* Hike 3) has entirely disappeared in the dense brush.

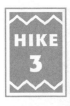

CASTAIC CREEK TO CIENAGA CAMPGROUND, FISH CANYON NARROWS, LION TRAIL CAMP

HIKE LENGTH: 17 miles round-trip; 1,600' elevation gain
DIFFICULTY: Moderate (2 days)
SEASON: All year
TOPO MAPS: *Whitaker Peak, Liebre Mountain, Burnt Peak*

Features

The long, shallow, meandering canyons in the northwest corner of Angeles National Forest are almost all laden with asphalt ribbon. One exception, and perhaps the most scenic canyon of them all, is Fish Canyon, which runs south from Sawmill Mountain, and then southwest into the Castaic Creek drainage.

Fish Canyon offers the best hiking in this part of the Angeles. An all-year stream descends its length, shaded most of the way by clusters of oaks, sycamores, alders, and willows. Most of the canyon is open and gently sloped—except for the 0.5-mile stretch of Fish Canyon Narrows, a slot through the mountain sometimes only a few yards wide. Abrupt, towering sidewalls of colorful rock make these narrows the most spectacular in the range—a Grand Canyon in miniature.

This very pleasant, almost level streamside trip ascends Fish Canyon from Castaic Creek; follows a dirt road to the Pianobox, an old mining prospect; passes through the scenic narrows to Rogers Trail Camp; and continues through the upper canyon to the delightful backcountry campsite of Lion Trail Camp. Be sure to wear stout and waterproof boots for the many stream crossings. This trip is best done as a two-day backpack outing, staying the night at either Rogers or Lion Camp.

Description

There is currently no vehicular access to the old trailhead at Cienaga Campground. Instead, you must now hike in, adding 5 miles round-trip to the total.

From I-5, 8 miles north of Castaic, turn east onto Templin Highway and follow it to where the road ends, blocked by a locked gate, a short distance from Castaic Creek. Park your car along the side of the road. Walk past the gate and continue down the highway, crossing the creek on a concrete bridge. Do not stray off the road or

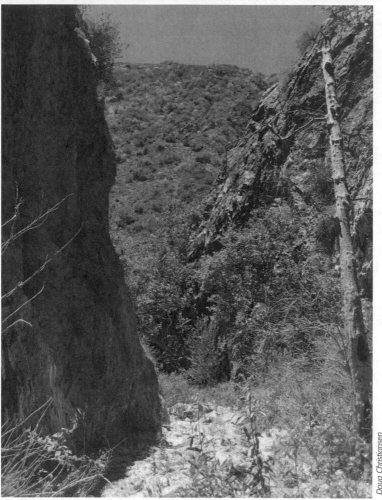

Fish Canyon Narrows

disturb private property. Be sure to display your Adventure Pass on your parked vehicle.

The road turns to dirt and continues eastward past the bridge; in a few hundred yards look for another dirt road branching off to the left. Follow this route as it heads north up the canyon along lower Fish Creek. Soon, the sidewalls close in and the scenery becomes lusher and greener, as the road—sometimes paved and sometimes dirt—crosses and recrosses Fish Creek several times. After walking 2.5 miles from your car, you come to open, parklike Cienaga Campground, located in a grove of oaks on a large flat along the creek.

From just north of Cienaga Campground, walk north, up Fish Creek, on any of the several jeep tracks. In 200 yards they converge into one dirt road, which you follow to the Pianobox, 1 mile from the campground.

From the Pianobox your trail follows the canyon as it turns northeast, and you abruptly enter the cool and shady narrows. Sheer sidewalls of reddish and yellowish rock make this area a favorite of shutter enthusiasts. Crossing and recrossing the stream, you work your way slowly up-canyon. In another mile you reach the oak- and sycamore-shaded bench of Rogers Camp, with stoves and tables. Just across the creek you can see a tunnel bored into solid rock, a relic of mining days. Beyond, the canyon rounds a bend, opens up, and resumes its northeast course. Your trail alternately follows the creek and climbs the slope to bypass narrows. Many sections of streamside trail are washed out, requiring much boulder-hopping and occasional bushwhacking. After 4 more difficult miles, 8.5 miles from your car, you reach Lion Trail Camp, located on an oak-shaded bench at the confluence of Lion and Fish Creeks. A stove, a fire ring, and a bench are here at this most isolated of Angeles Forest trail camps, a great spot to savor true wilderness away from the crowds that infest so much of the forest.

Return the same way. Or, you have another option. You can continue 4.5 miles up the Fish Canyon Trail, brushy in spots but passable, all the way to Atmore Meadows (*see* Hike 2). A less strenuous option is to hike this trail downhill, from Atmore Meadows to the Pianobox, necessitating a rather long car shuttle.

The Burnt Peak Canyon Trail, shown on the US Forest Service map, is, as of this writing, choked with brush and impassable.

The old trail from the Pianobox over the shoulder of Redrock Mountain to Redrock Canyon is no longer maintained by the US Forest Service and is badly overgrown. So the once-popular 24-mile circle backpack trip up Fish Canyon and over the ridge to Bear Canyon, down Bear, Cienaga, and Redrock Canyons is no longer an option.

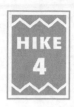

BOUQUET CANYON TO BIG OAK SPRING, SIERRA PELONA

HIKE LENGTH: 7 miles round-trip; 1,300' elevation gain
DIFFICULTY: Moderate
SEASON: All year
TOPO MAP: *Sleepy Valley*

Features

The Sierra Pelona—bare-topped, wind-buffeted, and lonely—forms a long arc across the northern mountains, separating Mint Canyon from first Bouquet Canyon and then Antelope Valley. Standing athwart the great wind funnel of Soledad Canyon, the crest is often battered by hurricane-force gusts. Sierra Pelona Lookout has recorded velocities of up to 100 miles per hour.

Nestled in protected recesses on the north slope of Sierra Pelona are isolated groves of live oaks, some of them patriarchal in stature. According to the American Forestry Association's Big Tree Register, the world's largest recorded canyon live oak—measuring 37 feet, 4 inches in trunk circumference—stands in a shallow draw on this north slope. Unfortunately, the tree was severely damaged in a brush fire many years ago. Today only its burned hulk remains, stark fingers pointing skyward.

This trip follows the Pacific Crest Trail up from Bouquet Canyon, visits Big Oak Spring and the charred remains of the world-record oak, and climbs to the top of Sierra Pelona for far-reaching vistas. Do it in summer, fall, winter, or spring—but not on a windy day.

Description

From Antelope Valley Freeway (CA 14), turn west onto Palmdale Boulevard, which becomes Elizabeth Lake Road. Follow it 9 miles, and then turn left (south) on Bouquet Canyon Road, following it 5 miles to the Pacific Crest Trail crossing. Park in the clearing to your left (south). Be sure to display your Adventure Pass on your parked vehicle.

Proceed up the signed PCT, climbing the north slope of chaparral-coated Sierra Pelona. As you gain altitude, you look down Bouquet Canyon, pastoral with its ranch houses and spreading oaks, with Bouquet Reservoir occasionally visible in the distance. You cross a poor jeep road and drop briefly into the upper reaches of Martindale Canyon before climbing again in a westward direction to a junction with the Big Oak Spring Trail, 2 miles from the start. Leave the PCT and follow the unimproved side trail through a grove of fire-damaged oaks. In about 200 yards you round a point and see the remains of the champion oak up to your left. A distinct pathway climbs to Big Oak Spring, a trickle of water guarded by stinging nettles (painful if they penetrate the skin). Return to the junction and continue up the PCT, now climbing southward, to the bare crest of Sierra Pelona, 1.5 more miles. Your vista now is impressive, especially if you walk a short distance west along the ridgetop fire road. Southeast, across the broad trench of Soledad Canyon, are the peaks of the main range— Mounts Gleason, Pacifico, Waterman, and Williamson. Northwest are the long hogbacks of Liebre and Sawmill Mountains. And north is the desert—sprawling, sun-bleached, and seemingly endless.

An option is to walk 3 miles east along the ridgetop fire road to Mount McDill (5,187') for an even better view. Descend the way you came. If you don't mind bushwhacking, you can drop down the old Big Tree Trail, its upper end 50 yards east of the Big Oak Spring Trail, to Bouquet Canyon Road, and then walk 0.5 mile east along the highway to your car. This trail has not been maintained in recent years.

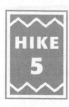

PLACERITA CANYON STATE PARK TO WALKER RANCH CAMPGROUND, LOS PINETOS SPRING, LOS PINETOS RIDGE, FIREBREAK RIDGE, MANZANITA MOUNTAIN

HIKE 5

HIKE LENGTH: 8 miles round-trip; 1,800' elevation gain
DIFFICULTY: Moderate
SEASON: October–June
TOPO MAPS: *Mint Canyon, San Fernando*

Features

Gentle hills, rounded ridgetops, oak-dotted canyons, and lots of chaparral—this describes the Placerita Canyon country near the western extremity of the main body of the San Gabriels. If you like your mountains simple, almost pastoral, and much less abrupt than usual for the San Gabriels, this is a trip for you.

Placerita Canyon is etched in history. California's first gold rush occurred here in 1842, six years before John Marshall's famous discovery at Coloma. It began when Francisco Lopez of Rancho San Francisco (near present-day Newhall) grew tired of chasing stray horses and sat down to rest under an oak tree. While resting, Lopez dug up a cluster of wild onions. Clinging to the roots were tiny gold nuggets. The discovery caused much excitement and attracted miners from all over California. These San Fernando Placers, as they become known, produced several hundred thousand dollars in gold before the excitement died down a few years later.

Today the gold rush area is preserved as Placerita Canyon State Park. The spot where Lopez is believed to have dug up the gold-bearing onions is known as "The Oak of the Golden Dream." It is marked with a plaque.

This trip goes up Placerita Canyon, shaded by overarching oaks and sycamores and graced with a trickling creek, to Walker Ranch Campground, and then climbs through chaparral and oaks to Los Pinetos Spring and on to the crest of Los Pinetos Ridge. Here, you are rewarded with far-reaching vistas north across the peaceful Placerita and Sand Canyon country, and southward across sprawling San Fernando Valley. Then you descend via the Firebreak Ridge–Manzanita Mountain Trail to complete a delightful loop hike.

Description

From the Antelope Valley Freeway (CA 14), turn right (east) onto Placerita Canyon Road and follow it 2 miles to Placerita Canyon State Park. Note that park hours are sunrise–sunset. Plan accordingly. Park in the easternmost dirt parking area to your right, just before the nature center.

Cross the creek and pick up the Walker Ranch Trail, marked by a wooden sign and metal pole, which leads east, on the right side of the creek. Follow the trail 2 miles as it winds its way up-canyon, crossing and recrossing the creek (with water in spring, but usually dry by midsummer) to Walker Ranch Group Campground. Here, you reach a three-way trail junction. The left trail goes 0.25 mile up to Placerita Canyon Road, an alternate trailhead. The path angling to your right is the Waterfall Trail, going up Los Pinetos Canyon 0.5 mile to a small cataract. On this trip you turn a sharp right (south) and follow the marked Los Pinetos Trail as it climbs the chaparral- and oak-coated west slope of Los Pinetos Canyon to Los Pinetos Spring, nestled in a woodsy recess, 2 miles from Walker Ranch Campground. Here, you meet a dirt road coming down from Los Pinetos Ridge fire road; don't take it. Just before the water tank, make a sharp right and follow the shortcut trail leading up to the ridgetop fire road, 0.5 mile.

If the day is hot, you may wish to return the way you came. There is no shade on the remainder of the loop trip. If the day is cool and you wish to continue, turn right (west) and follow the fire road uphill about 0.3 mile until you intersect the prominent firebreak leading north, down Firebreak Ridge. Turn right (north) and follow the firebreak as it descends north and then west, over several bumps, 2 miles to a junction with the trail leading right (north) down to Placerita Canyon State Park. (*Note:* You will see this trail to your right as you descend the last section of the firebreak; there is no sign at the junction, so watch for it carefully.) Descend the trail, passing a short side path left that leads 100 yards to the summit of Manzanita Mountain, to reach another junction just above the state park. Go right, passing a water tank, and descend a final 200 feet to the park. Cross Placerita Creek to your car.

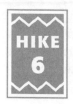

DILLON DIVIDE TO PACOIMA CANYON, DUTCH LOUIE FLAT, DAGGER FLAT

HIKE LENGTH: 6 miles round-trip; 800' elevation gain
DIFFICULTY: Moderate
SEASON: October–May
TOPO MAP: *Sunland*

Features

Rugged Pacoima Creek cuts a deep swath from the west slopes of Mount Gleason to the San Fernando Valley. An all-year stream rushes through the canyon bowels, shaded by oaks, cottonwoods, alders, and a handful of sycamores lower down. Dense chaparral clothes the north slope leading up to Santa Clara Divide, while the more protected south canyonside, below Mendenhall Ridge, is spotted with big-cone Douglas-firs. The 2009 Station Fire passed just east of here, sparing the riparian habitat along the stream as well as the surrounding slopes, and the canyon remains a sylvan delight.

Pacoima is derived from a Gabrielino word, possibly meaning "running water." American Indians once visited the lower canyon to gather acorns and hunt game. In more recent years, the canyon has been the scene of mining activities—for gold, silver, titanium, and graphite. Most notable were the G. C. K., or "Dutch Louie," placers; several thousand dollars in gold were recovered from the streambed. An old prospector known as Dutch Louie discovered the placers; to recover the gold, he and his associates diverted the stream by tunneling a temporary watercourse through a rock promontory. Today you can see the crumbling tunnel of this late-19th-century operation just upstream from Dutch Louie Flat. Three-quarters of a mile beyond, above Dagger Flat, are the remains of an old titanium mine.

This trip starts at Dillon Divide, drops down the dirt road into shady Pacoima Canyon to Dutch Louie Flat, and follows up the canyon, close by the sparkling creek, to Dagger Flat. Keep in mind that this is an "upside-down" hike—you finish with the 600-foot climb back up to the trailhead. Wear a good pair of proper hiking boots—there are several stream crossings where you must boulder-hop, and, if it's the wet season, plan on wading in two or three places.

Description

From the Foothill Freeway (I-210), just north of Hansen Dam, take the Osborne Street off-ramp. Follow Osborne Street north, with a short jog right at Foothill Boulevard, into Little Tujunga Canyon. Osborne becomes Little Tujunga Road; follow it 7.5 miles up to its intersection with gated Mendenhall Ridge Road (Forest Service Road 3N32) at Dillon Divide. Park to the right (north) of the highway without blocking the fire road. Be sure to display your Adventure Pass on your parked vehicle.

Pass the locked gate and follow dirt Mendenhall Ridge Road to a junction in 0.25 mile, go left and follow the dirt road down into Pacoima Canyon to Dutch Louie Flat (formerly a campground), 1.5 miles from Dillon Divide. Turn right and follow the eroded, rocky old road upstream as it disappears and reappears, crossing and recrossing the creek. In 0.25 mile you round a bend and see, to your left, the remains of the old Dutch Louie tunnel. Just beyond, along the creek, is where placer gold was once recovered. About 0.75 mile beyond is Dagger Flat, where a prospector was allegedly stabbed to death in the late 19th or early 20th century. From here, the old Dagger Flat Trail becomes overgrown and difficult to follow as it zigzags steeply up the north slope to Santa Clara Divide; don't take it—it's a shadeless bushwhack. You now have an option of lingering at Dagger Flat to check out the ghosts of the prospectors who once labored here for nature's elusive treasure, or of exploring a short distance farther up the canyon—it's mostly boulder-hopping from this point on. Return the way you came.

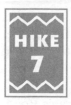

GOLD CREEK TO OAK SPRING, FASCINATION SPRING

HIKE 7

HIKE LENGTH: 8 miles round-trip; 2,000' elevation gain
DIFFICULTY: Moderate
SEASON: November–May
TOPO MAP: *Sunland*

Features

In the gentle hills above Little Tujunga Canyon are two delightful springs—little oak-sheltered recesses nestled in hills covered with chaparral. Both were largely spared by the 2009 Station Fire, although much of the surrounding slopes—particularly near and around Yerba Buena Ridge—burned. Oak Spring lies in a shallow recess near the head of Oak Spring Canyon, just over the ridge from Gold Creek. Fascination Spring—one can only guess how it got this intriguing name—is hidden in a narrow crease on the south slope of the mountains, 2,000 feet above the Sunland-Tujunga Valley.

You start from Gold Creek, Little Tujunga's major tributary. As the name suggests, Gold Creek was once the scene of feverish mining activity. Most storied were the so-called Little Nugget placers, recovering gold right from the creek bed. The gold is gone now, and this is ranch country.

A good trail leads south from Gold Creek and climbs into the gentle hill country of Yerba Buena Ridge. A mile and a half up is Oak Spring, hidden in a small draw so that you don't see it until you're almost there. Then you climb over Yerba Buena Ridge and drop abruptly down to Fascination Spring. The two springs are shaded by oaks; the rest of the trip is through open chaparral. This is an ideal outing for a cool winter or spring day. Try it after a rain, when the springs bubble full and the aroma of damp chaparral perfumes the clean air.

Description

From I-210 in Pacoima, just north of Hansen Dam, take the Osborne Street off-ramp. Go right onto Foothill Boulevard, and then immediately left on Osborne Street, which becomes Little Tujunga Road. Follow the latter 4 miles to Gold Creek Road. Turn right (east) and drive 0.75 mile to the marked Oak Springs Trailhead, on your right. Park in the oak-shaded clearing adjacent to the trailhead. Be sure to display your Adventure Pass on your parked vehicle.

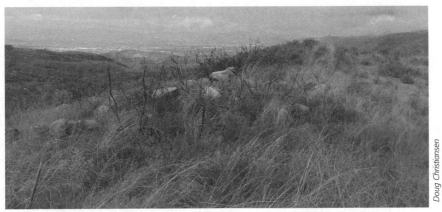

Doug Christiansen

Burned hillside above Fascination Spring

Proceed along the footpath across Gold Creek and up the chaparral-coated south slope. Follow the trail as it makes one long switchback, and then climbs south up the chaparral-covered hillside. Vistas open up over the wrinkled Gold Creek basin. The ranch you see down to the north is Paradise Ranch, scene of many a Cecil B. DeMille film extravaganza. Below to the east are the stone quarries where 770,000 tons of granite rock were removed for Hansen Dam in 1938–1940. In 1.25 miles you cross a divide and drop down to lush Oak Spring, where you'll find water except in the driest months. If it's a sunny day, the shade here is welcome. You may see a fire road coming down to Oak Spring from the other side; don't take it. Remain on the trail as it crosses the creek and contours around the slope (south). This section of trail isn't as good as what you've just been over, but it's easily passable. Follow the trail through dense chaparral and burn area from the Station Fire, around the slope, across a small gully, and up to the Yerba Buena Ridge fire road, 1.5 miles from Oak Spring. Here, you have a spectacular panorama southward over the Tujunga and San Fernando Valleys. Ignore the confusing trail signs here, which seem to point you in the wrong direction, and walk 100 yards down the road—toward the city—and then look carefully for the trail dropping south (left) down the steep mountainside. The pathway here is narrow and at times hard to follow as it contours around the slope in a generally southwest direction, follows a ridge, and then reverses course eastward. Fascination Spring lies nestled in a small gully, 1 mile from where you left the fire road and 900 feet lower in elevation.

Return the same way you came.

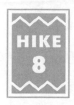

ALDER CREEK TO BARLEY FLATS

HIKE LENGTH: 7.5 miles round-trip; 2,100' elevation gain
DIFFICULTY: Moderate
SEASON: October–May
TOPO MAP: *Chilao Flat*

Features

Note: Barley Flats was heavily impacted by the 2009 Station Fire and as of this writing, spring 2013, remains closed to entry. Check with the US Forest Service to verify the current status of this area before attempting this hike.

Barley Flats is a prominent, forested ridge separating the watersheds of the Big Tujunga and West Fork. Not a true flats, it consists of a 2-mile-long rolling, forested plateau at an elevation of just over 5,000 feet.

The area has an interesting and varied past. As far back as the 1850s it was a well-known hideout for cattle rustlers and horse thieves, and it later became a favorite haunt of sportsmen and hunters. With the completion of the Shortcut Trail in 1893 (*see* Hike 53), Barley Flats was largely forgotten and fell into disuse. In the 1950s big changes arrived in the form of a Nike-Ajax antiaircraft missile site, one of several designed to serve as a defensive ring protecting the Los Angeles area. The administration buildings and facilities, still in good condition today, have served a variety of uses, functioning as a probation camp, search and rescue facility, and radio relay station.

You stand a good chance of having the trail to yourself; this Upper Big Tujunga–Alder Creek country is seldom traveled and is little known, having been largely bypassed by the Angeles Crest and Angeles Forest Highways. Don't do it on a hot day; the first portion of the route is shadeless and steep.

Description

From La Cañada, drive up Angeles Crest Highway to Clear Creek Junction. Turn left onto Angeles Forest Highway and follow it north, passing the Big Tujunga Canyon Road, to the junction with the *Upper* Big Tujunga Canyon Road. Turn right and follow it 4 miles to a dirt parking area along the right (south) side of the road, opposite a sign that says simply ALDER CREEK. Park along the highway. An alternate approach, from Foothill Boulevard in Sunland, is to drive up Oro

Vista Avenue, which becomes Big Tujunga Canyon Road, and follow it to its junction with Angeles Forest Highway, and then the Upper Big Tujunga Canyon Road. Be sure to display your Adventure Pass on your parked vehicle.

Walk down toward the creek bed and look for a metal pole; at this point cross the creek (dangerous after a major storm) and pick up the trail, overgrown in spots but passable, as it heads away from the creek and begins contouring up the chaparral-blanketed slopes. You soon come out onto a ridge and the trail steepens. Stop to rest often and enjoy the spectacular views, north into the Alder Creek drainage; east toward the rolling, forested Charlton Flat country; and west toward Strawberry Peak. After more steep climbing, you enter the welcome shade of a live oak forest, and continue for another mile through shady firs, Jeffrey pines, and Coulter pines to the paved Barley Flats Road, and the flats themselves, 3.7 miles from the start.

Return the way you came. With an 8-mile car shuttle between Alder Creek and Barley Flats, you can make it a one-way hike and halve the distance, starting at either end and hiking either uphill or downhill. The Barley Flats Road is located along Angeles Crest Highway, 4.9 miles past Red Box, just before the junction with the Upper Big Tujunga Canyon Road. Look for the trailhead near the end of the paved road, 2.7 miles from the Angeles Crest, and park along the side.

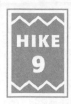

BIG TUJUNGA TO TOM LUCAS TRAIL CAMP, BIG CIENAGA

HIKE LENGTH: 8 miles round-trip; 2,000' elevation gain
DIFFICULTY: Moderate
SEASON: November–June
TOPO MAPS: *Sunland, Condor Peak*

Features

Trail Canyon cuts a deep swath through the western front country of the San Gabriels. Steep, chaparral-blanketed ridges surround it on both sides, and the great arched head of Condor Peak looms high on the eastern skyline. The scenic highlight is Trail Canyon Falls, 2 miles up-canyon, a delicate ribbon of whitewater swishing 30 feet into a cool sanctuary of alders and ferns.

It is appropriate that the campground be named after Tom Lucas, one of the real pioneers of the Big Tujunga. "Barefoot Tom," as he was known to his mountain friends, was one of the first forest rangers in the old San Gabriel Timberland Reserve, a grizzly bear hunter, and in his later years a rancher at the old Ybarra Ranch in the Big Tujunga. He knew the mountain country as few others did.

The canyon was once a lush and verdant oasis, until the 2009 Station Fire blackened the steep slopes and burned away much of the streamside greenery. It reopened to access in spring 2012 but is still undergoing repair. As of this writing in spring 2013, the trail is passable, but check with the US Forest Service to verify current conditions before attempting this hike. Note that Tom Lucas Trail Camp is closed pending repairs.

Description

From Foothill Boulevard in Sunland, drive 5 miles up Mount Gleason Avenue, which turns into Big Tujunga Canyon Road, to Upper Trail Canyon Road just prior to highway mileage marker 2.05. Turn left and drive up the winding dirt road to a junction, and then go right and down into Trail Canyon to a parking area beneath live oaks. Be sure to display your Adventure Pass on your parked vehicle.

Walk past the locked gate and follow the dirt road, passing some private cabins and crossing the creek on some well-placed planks. The old road climbs the east slope, then drops steeply back into the canyon, and ends. Ford the creek and pick up the trail as it threads its way up the boulder-filled canyon, crossing and recrossing the creek in foot-wetting fords. In 1 mile you reach a large, open bench on the left (west) side of the creek. Here, your trail leaves the creek and switch-backs steeply up to the left, and then climbs steadily up the slope to get around Trail Canyon Falls. In another 0.5 mile you round a sharp turn and then another turn, where the falls come into view, impressive as they plunge into the canyon depths below you. Just beyond where the trail again turns north, you will notice a narrow side path through the brush on which hikers have descended to the falls—very steep and loose footing. Continuing on the main trail, you drop back into the canyon above the falls and ford the creek again. Over the next 2 miles you follow the creek up-canyon, fording the stream several times, making your way around and through boulder fields, and reaching the old Tom Lucas campsite, no longer maintained by the US Forest Service. A mile beyond, where the canyon bends northward, your trail switchbacks up the slope, reapproaches the creek, crosses it, and reaches the new Tom Lucas Trail Camp—closed as of this writing in spring 2013—with picnic tables and cleared camping areas amid alders and oaks, 4 miles from the start. This area at the head of Trail Canyon Creek is known as Big Cienaga.

From the new Tom Lucas Trail Camp, the trail climbs, with several long switchbacks, to a branch of the Mendenhall Ridge fire road (*see* Hike 10), but you turn back at Big Cienaga.

As always, as you stroll down-canyon on the return trip, new vistas open up and you get a different perspective of the country. Most impressive, as you get back into the lower canyon, is the great buttress of Mount Lukens, towering on the southern skyline. This front-range country may be tamed and overrun by man, but it retains its rugged appeal. If it's late afternoon, chances are that a purplish haze will be adding a mystical quality to the mountain landscape. Mount Lukens may be a shadowy ghost in the distance.

A scenic option, 14 miles altogether, is to follow the Trail Canyon Trail up to its end at the spur road southeast of Iron Mountain, follow the spur road to the main Mendenhall fire road, turn left (west) and follow the fire road 3 miles to the Yerba Buena Trail, descend the trail to Gold Creek Saddle, 2 miles, and then descend the Gold Canyon fire road to Upper Trail Canyon road and follow the road down to your car. Check with the US Forest Service before attempting this route.

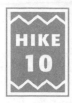

BIG TUJUNGA TO TOM LUCAS TRAIL CAMP, INDIAN BEN SADDLE, UPPER PACOIMA CANYON, DEER SPRINGS, MESSENGER FLATS CAMPGROUND

HIKE
10

HIKE LENGTH: 11 miles one way; 4,200' elevation gain
DIFFICULTY: Strenuous (1 day); moderate (2 days)
SEASON: May–October
TOPO MAPS: *Sunland, Condor Peak, Acton*

Features

Note: The Big Tujunga region was heavily impacted by the 2009 Station Fire and has only recently—spring 2012—been reopened to access. As of this writing in spring 2013, the trail is passable to Tom Lucas Trail Camp, but be sure to ask the US Forest Service about current conditions before venturing farther.

This delightful one-way trip (a car shuttle is recommended) climbs all the way up Trail Canyon to Mendenhall Ridge, and then ascends Upper Pacoima Canyon to Deer Springs and the pine-shaded Messenger Flats Campground just below Mount Gleason. You get superb views over the chaparral-clad and pine-dotted high country at the west end of the San Gabriels. You should be particularly delighted with the new trail stretch in Upper Pacoima, a canyon oasis of big-cone Douglas-firs, ponderosas, and sugar pines seldom trod by hikers.

This trip is best done as an overnight backpack, camping at Tom Lucas Trail Camp a third of the way up. The campground was severely damaged in the Station Fire and is undergoing repair; check ahead for the latest conditions if you plan to stay the night. You can do it in one long day, if you're a glutton for punishment. Unless you want to return the same long way and double your mileage, have someone meet you at Messenger Flats Campground, a 12-mile drive up Mount Gleason Road from Mill Creek Summit on the Angeles Forest Highway. Check with the US Forest Service to be sure the road is open; the gate on the road is sometimes closed. Bring a water bottle; there is all-year water in Trail Canyon and Upper Pacoima, but none in the open 3-mile stretch over Mendenhall Ridge and Indian Ben Saddle. Keep an eye on the weather: the 6,100-foot Messenger Flats Campground is sometimes closed by snow as late as May.

Description

From Foothill Boulevard in Sunland, drive 5 miles up Mount Gleason Avenue, which turns into Big Tujunga Canyon Road, to Upper Trail Canyon Road, just prior to highway mileage marker 2.05. Turn left and drive up the winding dirt road to a junction, and then go right and down into Trail Canyon to a parking area beneath live oaks. Be sure to display your Adventure Pass on your parked vehicle.

To get to the Messenger Flats Campground, where you should be picked up, drive up the Angeles Crest Highway to Clear Creek Junction, and then left up the Angeles Forest Highway (County Road N3) to Mill Creek Summit, 23 miles from La Cañada. Turn left (west) onto Mount Gleason Road—sometimes closed—and follow it 12 miles to the campground. Be sure to display your Adventure Pass on your parked vehicle.

Walk 3.5 miles up Trail Canyon to Tom Lucas Trail Camp (*see* Hike 9 for trail description). Fill your water bottle here. Continue up the trail through the marshy stretch known as Big Cienaga. Just beyond, your trail leaves the tree-shaded canyon and climbs up chaparral-blanketed slopes, passing a junction with the Condor Peak Trail, to a ridgetop where it meets a spur of the Mendenhall Ridge fire road. Follow the spur road and then the main fire road to Indian Ben Saddle (named for a gold prospector during depression days). Here, you pick up the new Upper Pacoima Trail leading northeast into the canyon. Follow the trail as it contours and then drops to the forested bottom of Pacoima Canyon and follows the creek some 2 miles before switchbacking up to Deer Spring. Go left at a trail junction there and follow the new path 1 mile to Messenger Flats Campground. (The trail to the right at Deer Springs goes 0.5 mile up to Lightning Point Group Campground; camping here is by reservation only.)

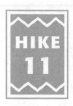

BIG TUJUNGA TO MOUNT LUKENS VIA STONE CANYON TRAIL

HIKE 11

HIKE LENGTH: 8 miles round-trip; 3,200' elevation gain
DIFFICULTY: Moderate
SEASON: November–May
TOPO MAP: *Condor Peak*

Features

Mount Lukens, a massive hogback mountain, lies just within the boundaries of Los Angeles, making it the highest point in the city. Years ago it was known as Sister Elsie Peak to commemorate the good deeds of a Roman Catholic nun in the La Crescenta Valley. Sister Elsie, in charge of El Rancho de Dos Hermanas orphanage for American Indian children, was much loved for her kind acts, particularly for nursing victims of a smallpox epidemic, during which she is reported to have lost her life. In the 1920s the US Forest Service renamed the peak Mount Lukens in honor of Theodore P. Lukens, one-time Angeles National Forest supervisor, famed for his reforestation efforts at Henninger Flat. A fire lookout was built on the summit in 1923; in 1937 it was moved to nearby Josephine Peak because, even then, urban haze was interfering with observation.

This trip is the best and shortest way to climb Mount Lukens—the only way that is not via a long, monotonous fire road. But it is exceptionally steep. The old Stone Canyon Trail—not regularly maintained but readily passable—wastes no mileage in going from Big Tujunga to the summit; it proceeds right up the north slope, without a level stretch until you reach the summit ridge. You're on burned slopes—thanks to the Station Fire—much of the way, with an occasional big-cone Douglas-fir or two for welcome shade. Carry a water bottle; you pass a sluggish spring about halfway up, but the water is not dependable.

Description

From Foothill Boulevard in Sunland, drive 6 miles up Mount Gleason Avenue, which becomes Big Tujunga Canyon Road, to its intersection with Doske Road; a sign says WILDWOOD PICNIC AREA. Before descending to the trailhead parking lot you may want to drive a short distance farther along the highway—several turnouts offer excellent vantage points from which your route across the Big Tujunga and beyond is clearly visible. From the intersection, turn right and

descend Doske Road to Stonyvale Road along the canyon bottom.
Turn left (upstream) on Stonyvale Road and drive about 0.5 mile to
the parking area at the end of the road. Walk past the end of the parking area and pick up the signed trail that crosses the stream. Be sure
to display your Adventure Pass on your parked vehicle.

Cross the Big Tujunga—difficult if not impossible when the water
is high—and head toward the trail on a sloping bench left (east) of
Stone Canyon Creek. Once you locate the trail, there's no problem.
Follow it as it zigzags steeply up the ridge left of Stone Canyon. In
about 2 miles you pass a small spring—a trickle of water during rainy
season. In 3.5 miles you reach an old fire road on the ridge northwest
of the summit. Turn left (southeast) and follow the bare path 0.25
mile to the top.

After enjoying the spectacular vista of the front-range country and
the city (if the smog isn't too bad), return the way you came. Or,
you can continue southeast and descend the long fire road and Dark
Canyon Trail to the Angeles Crest Highway (*see* Hike 13). This latter
option requires a car shuttle.

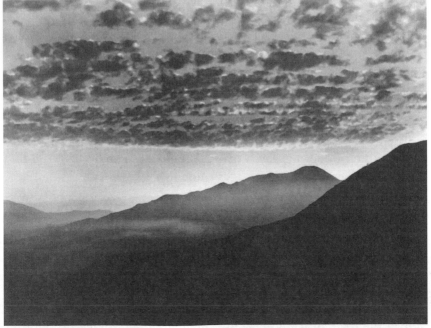

Huntington Library

Sunset over Mount Lukens

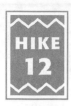

BIG TUJUNGA TO CONDOR PEAK VIA FOX DIVIDE

HIKE LENGTH: 16 miles round-trip; 3,400' elevation gain
DIFFICULTY: Strenuous
SEASON: November–May
TOPO MAP: *Condor Peak*

Features

Note: Check with the US Forest Service for up-to-date conditions before attempting this hike. The 2009 Station Fire decimated the Big Tujunga, and trail restoration and repairs are still ongoing.

There are no condors on Condor Peak, nor anywhere else in the San Gabriels today. The nearest redoubt of these magnificent birds is in the Sespe Creek area of Los Padres National Forest, some 50 miles northwest. Years ago, before humans disturbed its fragile habitat, this fast-vanishing species was common in all the Southern California mountains. According to mountain pioneer Faust Havermale, Condor Peak was so named because these monarchs of the air once nested here. Havermale wrote that he personally sighted 12 of these giant birds soaring around the peak, in the early 20th century.

But nostalgia for the departed birds is not the only reason for climbing Condor Peak. From its airy summit, you get a breathtaking panorama over the rugged Big Tujunga country and beyond to the major peaks of the front range—Lukens to the south and Josephine, Strawberry, and San Gabriel to the southeast. The mile-high atmosphere is fresh, clean, and invigorating.

There is no shade on the entire route, so the trip should be done on a cool winter or spring day. Carry all the water you'll need; the one water source en route is not always flowing.

Description

From Foothill Boulevard in Sunland, drive up Mount Gleason Avenue, which turns into Big Tujunga Canyon Road. In 7.25 miles you reach a parking area opposite the Vogel Flat Road intersection, where the trail begins. Be sure to display your Adventure Pass on your parked vehicle.

Walk about 150 yards up the highway to a small culvert on the left side of the road, near highway mileage marker 4.50. Pick up the trail where it enters the chaparral, and then bear right up the slope, cross a low ridge, and drop, and then contour and finally climb around a small canyon just above the highway.

For 3 miles, the trail zigzags up the divide between Vogel and Fusier Canyons, traverses a slope, passes a small creek (which usually has water in springtime), and finally reaches the high ridge between the head of Vogel Canyon and Fox Creek. You climb steeply, and then contour around the west side of Fox Peak before ascending the ridgetop firebreak over three false summits to the true summit of Condor Peak (5,439').

Descend by the same route. Or, with a 3-mile car shuttle, you can drop down the north slope of Condor Peak and follow the new trail north to its intersection with the Trail Canyon Trail, and then descend the latter to Big Tujunga (*see* Hike 9). You can also use this route to climb the peak.

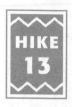

ANGELES CREST HIGHWAY TO GRIZZLY FLAT AND VASQUEZ CREEK

HIKE LENGTH: 4.5 miles round-trip; 1,100' elevation gain
DIFFICULTY: Easy
SEASON: November–May
TOPO MAP: *Condor Peak*

Features

Note: As with all hikes in the Station Fire burn area, check with the US Forest Service to verify current conditions before attempting this hike. The area traversed by this trip was only recently reopened to hikers, and although passable, the trail is still in need of more reworking and repair.

Grizzly Flat is a rather conspicuous sloping bench on the mountainside south of Big Tujunga, directly above where the great canyon elbows northeast. The flat is cut abruptly on both sides—on the west by an unnamed gully and on the east by fir-shaded Vasquez Creek. There was once a healthy forest here, but fire burned most of it away in 1959 and again in 2009. What humans destroy in a careless instant, nature takes years to rebuild.

Grizzly Flat, Vasquez Creek—these names bring to mind two scourges of the San Gabriels of yesteryear: grizzly bears and bandidos.

Grizzlies once abounded in these mountains, and old-timers' recollections are full of exciting encounters with these forest behemoths, which seemed to favor the Big Tujunga region particularly. The last verified grizzly bear south of the Tehachapis was killed in lower Big Tujunga in 1916.

Vasquez Creek immortalizes an 1874 foray by Southern California's most famous bandit, Tiburcio Vásquez. After raiding the Repetto Ranch, in the hills south of San Gabriel Valley, Vásquez and his small gang took off with $500, hotly pursued by a sheriff's posse. The outlaws hurried up the Arroyo Seco, ascended Dark Canyon to the divide, and dropped down an unnamed creek into Big Tujunga. The posse, guessing that Vásquez was heading for Big Tujunga, backtracked and raced around to the canyon entrance to block his escape. But the bandidos, urging their horses to the limit, just managed to race out of the canyon ahead of the converging lawmen. Since this episode, the stream in the gully, down which the bandits descended to Big Tujunga, has been known as Vasquez Creek.

Description

Drive up the Angeles Crest Highway 6.1 miles from La Cañada to a small parking area (big enough for four or five cars) opposite highway mileage marker 30.02. Be sure to display your Adventure Pass on your parked vehicle.

The 0.5-mile trail begins at the lower (south) end of the parking area and climbs steeply up the slope to a loop road at the lower edge of a tree plantation—mostly burned now. Go right and follow the dirt road up to fire road 2N80 on the crest of the divide between the Arroyo Seco and Big Tujunga watersheds. Cross 2N80 and descend an unmarked dirt road to Grizzly Flat, amid a grove of pines—heavily damaged in the Station Fire—planted by the US Forest Service after a previous fire in 1959. A faint, unmarked trail goes right (northeast) to Vasquez Creek, 0.25 mile away. There is no trail along Vasquez Creek, but you can follow the creek a short distance in either direction.

With a car shuttle, you can follow the 3-mile trail northwest from Grizzly Flat, crossing a small unnamed creek, down to Big Tujunga Creek, which you must ford, and on to Stonyvale Picnic Area. See Hike 11 for the driving route (Stonyvale Picnic Area is just beyond the Stone Canyon Trailhead). Avoid this alternative after heavy rains; Big Tujunga swells to a raging torrent.

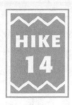

TUJUNGA TO MOUNT LUKENS VIA HAINES CANYON TRAIL

HIKE LENGTH: 8 miles round-trip; 2,800' elevation gain
DIFFICULTY: Moderate
SEASON: November–May
TOPO MAP: *Condor Peak*

Features

This is the old Sister Elsie Trail up the southwest shoulder of Mount Lukens, eventually linking up with the Stone Canyon Trail (*see* Hike 11). There is little shade en route, so do it on a cool winter or spring day. Check with the US Forest Service for up-to-date trail conditions; the trip passes through the 2009 Station Fire burn area and has only recently, as of this writing, been reopened.

Description

From Foothill Boulevard in Tujunga, go north on Haines Canyon Avenue, jogging a half block east at Day Street. Continue up Haines Canyon Avenue to the locked gate just short of the debris dam. Park along the road, being careful to observe parking restrictions. Apperson Street has additional parking.

Walk up the road beyond the gate. Stay on the main road, ignoring any turnoffs, until, at 1.5 miles from the trailhead, the road turns right and begins to climb the south canyon slope. Just short of this point look for a narrow, unmarked trail that branches off to the left. Follow this path up-canyon as it passes a cement water tank, narrows, and at 0.75 mile from the road junction reaches another junction— just short of a stream crossing. Continue straight ahead, crossing the creek. (The trail to the right switchbacks up the canyon wall and joins the fire road halfway to the summit.) Your trail becomes increasingly indistinct as you follow the canyon bottom another 0.5 mile, and then turn right and zigzag up a steep side canyon. Here, you are in oak woodland—mostly spared by the 2009 Station Fire. In 0.5 mile, near the canyon head, your trail abruptly zigs left and reaches a saddle on Mount Lukens's west ridge, where views open northward across the mighty gorge of Big Tujunga. You climb along the ridgetop for 0.25 mile, and then contour left along the steep north slope of the ridge to a junction with the Stone Canyon Trail (*see* Hike 11). Follow the latter, and then follow the fire road to the summit.

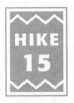

ALTADENA TO OAKWILDE VIA ARROYO SECO

HIKE LENGTH: 9 miles round-trip; 900' elevation gain
DIFFICULTY: Moderate
SEASON: November–May
TOPO MAP: *Pasadena*

Features

Note: Although most of the streamside habitat was spared, the 2009 Station Fire decimated the surrounding mountainsides. The Arroyo Seco has only recently been reopened to hikers. The trail is currently, as of spring 2013, closed at Paul Little Memorial Picnic Area. With luck, the remainder of this historic pathway will soon be open, but check with the US Forest Service for the latest conditions.

Today the Arroyo Seco is largely bypassed and forgotten. Seventy years ago it was one of the most popular vacation spots in the range. Under its luxuriant cover of willows, sycamores, alders, and bays, the canyon reverberated with the lusty shouts and merry songs of hikers and campers. The lower reaches were dotted with rustic cabins and well-used picnic spots. This was before the Angeles Crest Highway provided ready access into the mountains, climbing high on the west slope of the canyon. Now nature's stillness reigns supreme in the canyon, broken only by the gentle murmur of the stream, the soft rustle of sycamore leaves, and—as a reminder of civilization's nearness—the occasional muffled roar of an automobile rounding a curve far above.

About halfway up this great gorge, on a forested streamside bench, is Oakwilde Picnic Area, with tables and stoves. Here, in 1911, J. R. Phillips fashioned a tourist resort, old Camp Oak Wilde. For almost three decades, until it was nearly obliterated in the 1938 flood, this was a favorite spot of vacationing Southlanders. In the 1920s a road was built up the lower Arroyo Seco to the camp; it, too, was severely damaged in the greatest torrent ever known in the San Gabriels. Today only remnants of the road remain, and a few stone foundations at Oakwilde are the only signs of what once went on here.

Time and nature's gradual healing process have restored much of the beauty of the Arroyo Seco. Although parts of the lower canyon have been permanently marred by man's work—most notably the Brown Canyon Debris Dam—there is much to be seen and enjoyed in this great canyon; this trail trip gives you a fair sampling.

Description

From I-210, take the Arroyo Boulevard off-ramp and drive north on Arroyo, which promptly becomes Windsor Avenue. Continue north 0.75 mile to the intersection with Ventura Street.

You will notice two roads—both with gates usually locked—leading north down toward the canyon entrance. Take the right (eastern) of the two; the left road goes to the Jet Propulsion Laboratory parking lot. Proceed on foot down the road, which gains the Arroyo Seco entrance in 0.5 mile. You pass the assorted markings of the Pasadena Water Department—fences, retaining walls, gauging stations, and a host of warning signs—and reach US Forest Service residences in another 0.5 mile. Go left at a road fork; now, the canyon closes in and the scenery becomes more woodsy—giant canyon oaks, alders, willows, sycamores, and even a few eucalyptus trees from resort days. This is both a hiking and an equestrian route, so you'll most likely pass horseback riders. The trail alternates between following the old road and stream-hopping where the roadbed and bridges have washed out.

A half mile above the US Forest Service residences is Teddy's Outpost Picnic Area—named for a small roadside resort operated by Theodore "Teddy" Syvertson from 1914 to 1926. In another 0.5 mile you reach the Gould Mesa Campground, honoring Will Gould, who homesteaded here in the 1890s, and just beyond, a side road leading up to Gould Mesa and the Angeles Crest Highway. Nino Picnic Area is 0.3 mile farther. Above Nino the canyon narrows, twists, and turns, and remnants of the old road become less evident. In another 0.75 mile you reach Paul Little Memorial Picnic Area, 100 feet to your left. Going right, the trail climbs up the steep east slope of the canyon to get around Brown Canyon Debris Dam, and then drops back into the gorge and rounds two sharp bends before reaching Oakwilde, 4.5 miles from the start. Here, amid the crumbling foundations of the old road's-end resort, under live oaks and alders, the US Forest Service has built Oakwilde Trail Camp, with tables and stoves.

Return the way you came.

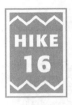

ANGELES CREST HIGHWAY TO OAKWILDE, ARROYO SECO, SWITZER TRAIL CAMP, AND SWITZER'S PICNIC AREA

HIKE LENGTH: 10.5 miles one way; 1,500' elevation gain
DIFFICULTY: Moderate
SEASON: November–May
TOPO MAPS: *Condor Peak, Pasadena*

Features

Note: As of this writing, spring 2013, the majority of this hike lies within the Station Fire Recovery Area. The Arroyo Seco is open only from the Altadena trailhead to Paul Little Memorial Picnic Area (*see* Hike 15) and in the vicinity of Switzer's (*see* Hike 17). Check ahead with the US Forest Service to verify the status of this hike before attempting.

This trip drops into the Arroyo Seco from high on the Angeles Crest Highway, and then traverses the wild central portion of the Arroyo Seco Trail to Switzer Trail Camp. En route it passes through the sites of two once-famous mountain resorts—Oak Wilde and Switzer's Camp. To avoid the difficult middle gorge of the Arroyo Seco, known as Royal Gorge to old-timers, the trail climbs up and over chaparral-blanketed ridges, which are not very pleasant to walk on a hot day. Do it when the weather is cool. A car shuttle is required.

Description

The historic Dark Canyon Trail is temporarily impassable because of a massive slide. Until the US Forest Service rebuilds the trail, hikers must use the paved fire road down into the Arroyo Seco from Gould Mesa. Drive from La Cañada up the Angeles Crest Highway 2 miles, just past the first big bend, near highway mileage marker 26.47, to a gated road on your right under a power line, where a small wooden sign points right (east) and indicates GABRIELINO TRAIL. Park in the clearing on your right just below the gated road. Be sure to display your Adventure Pass on your parked vehicle.

Proceed around the locked gate through a hikers' entrance to the right, and then follow the road east, passing a power substation on your right. Beyond the station, the road narrows and winds steeply down into the Arroyo Seco, where you intersect the Arroyo Seco Trail, 0.5 mile. Follow the trail upstream, crossing and recrossing the creek, climbing the east slope to pass the Brown Canyon Debris Dam, and then dropping back to the canyon floor and fording the creek once again to the Oakwilde Picnic Area, 3.5 miles from the start. Continue up the Arroyo Seco, fording and refording the stream (foot-wetting in times of high water). About a mile above Oakwilde the arroyo makes a sharp turn east and becomes a narrow gorge, difficult of passage. Here, the trail leaves the main canyon, ascends the east fork of Long Canyon, and climbs high over chaparral ridges before dropping back into the Arroyo Seco at Switzer Trail Camp, 3.5 miles from Oakwilde. Shaded by magnificent alders

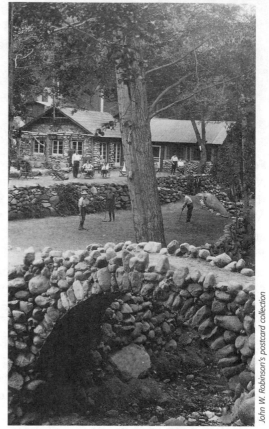

Switzer Camp (circa 1928)

and oaks, the most popular trail resort in the range once stood here (*see* Hike 17). Today the buildings are gone. A mile farther up-canyon, partly by boulder-hopping and partly on the remains of an old road, you reach spacious Switzer's Picnic Area and a paved road up to the Angeles Crest Highway.

As an alternative you can do this trip in reverse, starting at Switzer's Picnic Area and finishing on Gould Mesa—mostly downhill, with a 500-foot gain at the end.

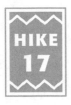

SWITZER'S PICNIC AREA TO COMMODORE SWITZER TRAIL CAMP, SWITZER FALLS, ARROYO SECO CASCADES

HIKE LENGTH: 4 miles round-trip;
600' elevation gain and loss
DIFFICULTY: Easy
SEASON: November–June
TOPO MAP: *Condor Peak*

Features

Once, the name Switzer was almost synonymous with Arroyo Seco. This was when Switzer Camp was the most famous trail resort in the range. By foot, by horse, or by burro, hundreds of people traveled up the Arroyo Seco every weekend to visit this picturesque, woodsy hostelry above Switzer Falls.

It was Commodore Perry Switzer—along with the mountain-loving Watermans, Bob and Liz—who fashioned this wilderness resort back in 1884. Twice weekly, Switzer led his burro train up the tortuous Arroyo Seco Trail, featuring 60 stream crossings and endless switchbacks. A cow horn was left dangling on a manzanita bush 0.5 mile below camp, with printed instructions to issue forth a blast for each hungry guest. When the tired visitors finally reached camp, they would find a sizzling dinner awaiting them. Trout from the adjacent stream were featured.

It was under hospitable Lloyd and Bertha Austin (1912–1936) that Switzer's really became the number one resort in the range. The warmth and friendliness of the Austins attracted thousands from all walks of life. Among those who signed the guest register were Henry Ford, Shirley Temple, Clark Gable, and Mary Pickford. LEAVE YOUR CARES AND ANIMALS THIS SIDE OF THE STREAM was the sign that greeted approaching visitors; another sign over the lodge door read THE AUSTIN HOME . . . AND YOURS. So that his guests would have the opportunity for a variety of experiences, Austin added a tennis court, a croquet court, a well-stocked library, a children's playground, an open-air dance floor for Switzer Saturday Nights, and a miniature Christ Chapel perched above the falls for Sunday morning worship.

All this is gone now, the victim of progress in the form of the Angeles Crest Highway. With people able to drive in minutes to places that once required hours or days of strenuous hiking, the old camp lost its wilderness appeal. After withering for two decades, it was finally abandoned and all buildings removed in 1959. Today the sylvan bench just above the falls is occupied by Commodore Switzer Trail Camp—a wilderness campsite with no facilities.

This trip is a delightful streamside stroll under alder, oak, maple, and sycamore trees. Though the Station Fire roared through here in 2009, the streamside habitat fared quite well. You visit the old campsite and then descend into the narrow Royal Gorge of the Arroyo Seco for a close-up view of plunging Switzer Falls

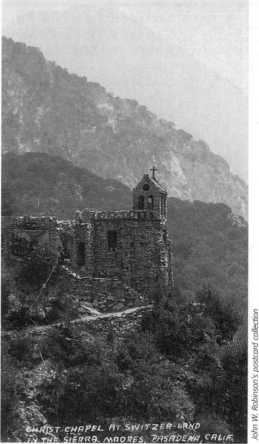

Switzer's Chapel (1924–1959)

John W. Robinson's postcard collection

and the numerous little pools and cascades that dot the shady chasm. (Don't try to climb the falls; several have been injured in the attempt.)

Description

Drive up the Angeles Crest Highway 10.5 miles from La Cañada to the side road down to Switzer's Picnic Area, 0.5 mile past the junction of the Angeles Crest and Angeles Forest Highways. Turn right and descend to the parking area outside the picnic area, 0.25 mile. Be sure to display your Adventure Pass on your parked vehicle.

Cross the bridge and follow the trail down-canyon. It is a mile to Commodore Switzer Trail Camp; part of the distance you must boulder-hop, where the trail is washed out. From the trail camp, cross the stream and follow the trail as it climbs and then contours along the west slope above the falls. Do *not* follow the creek below camp; it abruptly drops 50 feet at the falls. About 0.25 mile beyond camp is an unmarked junction: the right (southwest) fork is the main Arroyo Seco Trail—closed to access as of this writing in spring 2013—down to Oakwilde and Pasadena (*see* Hikes 15 and 16). Go left (southeast), dropping into the gorge of the Arroyo Seco below the falls. When you reach the creek, turn upstream 0.25 mile to Switzer Falls. Remember, don't climb the sheer rock sidewalls of the falls. Then turn back downstream and follow the woodsy gorge past numerous sparkling pools and miniature cascades, about a mile to the Bear Canyon junction. This secluded part of the Arroyo Seco is one of the most beautiful spots in the front range, beckoning to any who are willing to leave their automobile and stroll for a leisurely two or three hours.

Return the way you came.

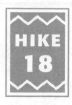

SWITZER'S PICNIC AREA TO COMMODORE SWITZER TRAIL CAMP, BEAR CANYON, BEAR CANYON TRAIL

HIKE 18

HIKE LENGTH: 8 miles round-trip; 1,000' elevation gain
DIFFICULTY: Moderate
SEASON: November–June
TOPO MAPS: *Condor Peak, Pasadena*

Features

Rugged Bear Canyon, the largest tributary of the Arroyo Seco, is as near to being wilderness as any place in the front range of the San Gabriels. A beautiful stream, with mirrorlike pools, cascades, and small waterfalls, graces the canyon bottom. Stately big-cone Douglas-firs keep much of the creek in near-perpetual shade. By a fortunate accident of geography, Bear Canyon is isolated from man's frenetic activity even though it lies smack in the middle of the much-abused front range. Although highways and fire roads virtually circle the chasm, none comes quite close enough to violate its sanctity.

This trip descends the Arroyo Seco to its junction with Bear Canyon, and then ascends the latter to lonely Bear Canyon Trail Camp, set on a shaded streamside bench about halfway up the canyon. You will be tempted to stay the night here, where nature retains a small foothold, and civilization—just over the ridge—seems far away.

Wear lug-soled boots; the old Tom Sloan Trail that once traveled the length of the canyon is in poor shape, and you must scramble and boulder-hop much of the way.

Description

Drive up the Angeles Crest Highway 10.5 miles from La Cañada to the side road down to Switzer's Picnic Area, 0.5 mile past the junction of the Angeles Crest and Angeles Forest Highways. Turn right and descend to the parking area outside the campground, 0.25 mile. Be sure to display your Adventure Pass on your parked vehicle.

Cross the bridge and follow the trail down-canyon, past Commodore Switzer Trail Camp, and down into the gorge of the Arroyo Seco below Switzer Falls (*see* Hike 17 for details). Continue down the Arroyo Seco gorge another 0.75 mile to the junction with Bear Canyon (2 miles from the start). The trail turns east up Bear Canyon, skipping from side to side. Frequently it disappears; continue along the creek and you will find it again. About 2 miles up the canyon, the trail climbs onto a forested bench on the south slope, about 20 feet above the stream. Here is Bear Canyon Trail Camp. Be on the lookout for this spot; it is easy to miss the trail leading up the slope.

This trip returns the same way. You also have the option of continuing up the canyon trail another 2 miles, and then steeply up to Tom Sloan Saddle and the Mount Lowe fire road (*see* Hike 33), or dropping from the saddle into Millard Canyon (*see* Hike 19). Either of these options requires a car shuttle. Note that as of this writing, spring 2013, this last route lies within the Station Fire Recovery Area and is closed to entry. Check ahead with the US Forest Service to verify the current status of this area.

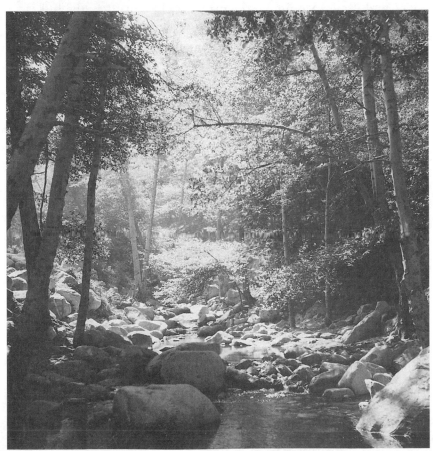

Arroyo Seco above Switzer Trail Camp

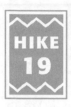

MILLARD CANYON TO DAWN MINE

HIKE LENGTH: 5 miles round-trip; 1,200' elevation gain
DIFFICULTY: Moderate
SEASON: November–May
TOPO MAP: *Pasadena*

Features

Note: Millard Canyon lies within the Station Fire Recovery Area and is, as of this writing (spring 2013), closed to entry. Check with the US Forest Service for updates before attempting this hike.

Woodsy Millard Canyon ranks as one of the more pleasant retreats in the front range of the San Gabriels. Nestled deep between Sunset Ridge and Brown Mountain, the canyon seldom suffers the full glare of sunlight. Beneath overarching oaks and sycamores, the small stream glides and dances over water-tempered boulders, finally to tumble headlong over Millard Falls.

Deep in the upper reaches of Millard Canyon are the remains of the Dawn Mine, the most storied gold prospect in the front range. Gold was discovered here in 1895, and the ore-bearing veins were worked on and off with varying degrees of success into the early 1950s. No great amount of gold was ever recovered, despite repeated boasts of imminent bonanzas by overoptimistic prospectors.

The trail up Millard Canyon to Dawn Mine is no longer maintained. In its middle and upper stretches, where it closely parallels the stream, it is almost gone, and boulder-hopping is the order of the day. But the canyon is a sylvan delight, where you can temporarily forget your proximity to civilization. It is a peaceful place to while away the hours, to saunter rather than stride.

Description

From Loma Alta Drive in Altadena, turn north on Chaney Trail Drive, pass through a gate—open 6 a.m.–8 p.m.—and follow it to the junction atop Sunset Ridge; turn right and park outside the locked gate blocking the Sunset Ridge fire road. Observe and heed the NO PARKING signs along the road. If you are here on the weekend and this small parking area is full, your best bet is to continue down to the bottom of Millard Canyon, another 0.5 mile. Be sure to display your Adventure Pass on your parked vehicle.

Hike up the Sunset Ridge fire road, where you will almost immediately see a trail that leads left; don't take it. Stay on the paved fire
road for another 300 yards to an intersection with the marked Sunset
Ridge Trail leading left. Follow this trail around the ridge and down
into Millard Canyon above the falls. Just before you reach the canyon
bottom, at a trail junction, go left (the right branch leads back up to
Sunset Ridge fire road). When the trail reaches the streambed, it all
but disappears in a jumble of boulders. As you scramble upstream,
you will occasionally meet stretches of the old trail, but mostly, you
will boulder-hop. After slightly more than a mile, the canyon suddenly elbows north; here, your route becomes more difficult until
you reach a series of massive boulders that bar any farther travel.
Look carefully along the left bank for a narrow use trail under a large
bay tree that climbs up and around this granite roadblock before
returning once again to the stream. As you continue upstream, stay
in the main canyon; do not take any of the small side canyons you
may see on the right. Less than a mile of additional boulder-hopping
brings you to the woodsy haunt that once was Dawn Mine. Not much
remains—scattered diggings, pieces of rusted mill machinery, and a
narrow tunnel entrance. Do not try to explore the tunnel; there are
water-filled holes difficult to detect. After looking over the shaded
sanctuary, return the way you came.

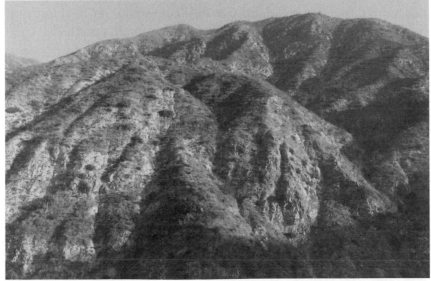

Burned mountainside above Millard Canyon

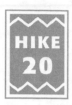

MILLARD CANYON TO MILLARD CANYON FALLS

HIKE LENGTH: 1 mile round-trip; 150' elevation gain
DIFFICULTY: Easy
SEASON: November–May
TOPO MAP: *Pasadena*

Features

Note: Access to the falls is closed due to the Station Fire. I hope this popular pathway will reopen in the near future. Check ahead with the US Forest Service to verify the current status of the trail.

Of the two dozen or so real waterfalls in the San Gabriel Mountains, only four are readily accessible to the leisurely stroller. Millard Canyon Falls is one of these. The 50-foot falls are wedged snugly where the lower canyon narrows, about 0.5 mile above the Millard Canyon picnic area. The short canyon-bottom walk is shaded most of the way by huge canyon oaks and a handful of tall alders and willows. Only a short distance from Altadena, this route makes an ideal Sunday-afternoon saunter.

Description

Drive up Chaney Trail Drive in Altadena. Note the gate that you pass through on your way up—it is closed 8 p.m.–6 a.m. Continue over the ridge and down to the parking area at the bottom of Millard Canyon. Be sure to display your Adventure Pass on your parked vehicle.

Pass a locked gate and proceed a hundred yards up the fire road to Millard Canyon Public Campground. At the upper end of the campground, a wooden sign points right (east) to Millard Canyon Falls. Follow the shady canyon trail 0.5 mile to the foot of the falls. Don't try to climb over the falls; people have been injured attempting this dangerous feat. Return the way you came.

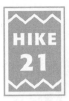

BROWN MOUNTAIN LOOP

HIKE LENGTH: 12 miles round-trip; 2,500' elevation gain
DIFFICULTY: Strenuous
SEASON: November–May
TOPO MAP: *Pasadena*

Features

Note: As of this writing, spring 2013, this trip lies within the Station Fire Recovery Area and is closed to entry. Check ahead with the US Forest Service for updates before attempting this hike.

The "Brown Boys"—Owen and Jason—were familiar figures in and around the foothills of the front range back in the 1880s. These long-bearded sons of fiery pre–Civil War abolitionist John Brown lived in a small log cabin near the head of El Prieto Canyon, a beautiful wooded glen between the Arroyo Seco and Millard Canyon. Great lovers of nature, the men spent much time exploring the neighboring mountains. They sought out a mountain peak to name in honor of their famous father. After an abortive attempt to place his name on what later became known as Mount Lowe, they settled on the long, rounded mountain rising high between Millard Canyon and Bear Creek. Today it is still known as Brown Mountain.

This lengthy loop trip climbs up Millard Canyon to Tom Sloan Saddle (named for a former district ranger), traverses the 4,485-foot hogback of Brown Mountain, and descends from the west ridge around the south slope

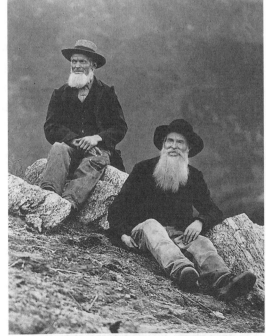

Owen and Jason Brown, two sons of John Brown, on Brown Mountain (circa 1884)

Huntington Library

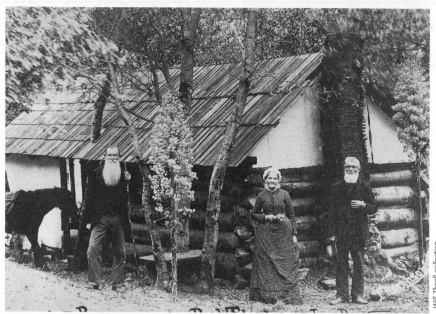

"Brown Boys" at their El Prieto Cabin (circa 1887)

back to the starting point. You should be in good physical condition for this one, and because part of the loop is trailless, wear lug-soled boots.

Description

From Loma Alta Drive in Altadena, turn north on Chaney Trail Drive and follow it through a gate—locked 8 p.m.–6 a.m.—to the junction atop Sunset Ridge; turn right and park outside the locked gate that blocks the Sunset Ridge fire road. If this small parking area is full, continue another 0.5 mile down to the bottom of Millard Canyon and park in the lot. Be sure to display your Adventure Pass on your parked vehicle.

Hike up the Sunset Ridge fire road about 400 yards to the signed Sunset Ridge Trail leading left, around the ridge into Millard Canyon above the falls (*see* Hike 19). Follow the streamside trail, hopping boulders where the footpath has been washed out, to the Dawn Mine. From the mine, cross the stream and follow a narrow trail that switchbacks up a small slope to a junction; go left and then almost immediately left again at another junction. Don't take the trail from this second fork that goes sharply to the right; it leads back up to the fire road. Follow the path north as it continues up-canyon to where the creek splits; take the left (west) fork and follow the creek along the left bank a very short distance and look for the trail on the right (east) bank. Follow this hard-to-spot pathway as it climbs out of the canyon and zigzags north up to Tom Sloan Saddle, 3.5 miles from the start. Here, you stand on the divide between Millard Canyon and Bear Creek, a three-way trail junction (*see* Hike 33). From the saddle, leave the trail and scramble left (west) up the firebreak and a faint hikers' footpath, climbing over or around three false summits, to the true hogback summit of Brown Mountain, slightly more than a mile.

Standing on the bare summit, you are rewarded with a superb panorama of the front range. To the west, across the yawning chasm of the Arroyo Seco, is Mount Lukens. Northward, beyond Bear Creek and the upper Arroyo Seco, are the impressive humps of Josephine and Strawberry Peaks. Eastward are the triumvirate of San Gabriel Peak, Mount Markham, and Mount Lowe. And to the south, past Millard Canyon, sprawls the megalopolis, usually half hidden in brown murkiness.

When you're through looking, continue west along the firebreak, dropping 1,600 feet in 2 miles to the upper end of the Brown Mountain fire road (closed to public vehicles). Proceed down the fire road as it curves southeastward around the lower slopes of Brown Mountain. Go left (east) at all road junctions. After 6 miles, the fire road reaches the Millard Canyon Public Campground. Because your car is up on Sunset Ridge (unless you arranged a car shuttle), you'll have to climb 400 feet up the other side of the canyon. At the lower end of the campground, take the unmarked trail that leads left from the fire road and climbs to the ridgetop just above the parking area.

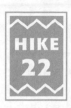

SUNSET RIDGE TO
MOUNT LOWE CAMPGROUND

HIKE LENGTH: 11 miles round-trip; 2,400' elevation gain
DIFFICULTY: Strenuous (1 day); moderate (2 days)
SEASON: November–May
TOPO MAPS: *Pasadena, Mount Wilson*

Features

The Mount Lowe Scenic Railway was one of the early 20th century's engineering marvels, visited by tens of thousands during its 43 years of operation (1893–1936). This trip climbs the Sunset Ridge Trail, above Millard Canyon, to the old railway bed near what was once called the Cape of Good Hope. The route then follows the railway bed, now the Sunset Ridge–Mount Lowe fire road, to the Mount Lowe Tavern site, presently Mount Lowe Trail Camp. The old railway bed is gently graded and offers a splendid panorama over mountain, canyon, and lowland—particularly on a clear winter or spring day when air pollution does not muddy the sky. You will pass some of the "stations" denoting historic sites on the old railroad, with signs and plaques erected by weekend volunteers of the Scenic Mount Lowe Railway Historical Committee. Most of the surrounding slopes were burned in the 2009 Station Fire; Millard Canyon itself, as of this writing, is still closed to access.

You can make this a strenuous one-day trip or stay overnight at Mount Lowe Trail Camp, making it a very pleasant two-day outing. *Note:* The water at Mount Lowe Trail Camp is, at this writing, unsafe for drinking without treatment. Check with the US Forest Service for the latest water condition.

Description

From Loma Alta Drive in Altadena, turn north on Chaney Trail Drive, drive through a gate—locked 8 p.m.–6 a.m.—and continue up to the ridgetop junction; turn right and park outside the locked gate blocking the Sunset Ridge fire road. Do not block the road. If the small parking area here is full, continue down to the parking lot at the bottom of the canyon, another 0.5 mile. Be sure to display your Adventure Pass on your parked vehicle.

Walk past the locked gate and up the fire road about 400 yards to a junction on your left. Take the signed Sunset Ridge Trail, which contours around the ridge above Millard Canyon. Just before you reach the canyon bottom is a trail junction. Go right (the left branch goes up Millard Canyon) and follow the trail all the way up to the top of Sunset Ridge, 2.5 miles, where you rejoin the fire road. As you proceed up the fire road, Echo Mountain and its historical ruins come into view down to your right. In 0.5 mile you meet the old railway bed coming up from Echo Mountain. Just beyond, you pass a metal post (the first of the "stations") on your left, indicating that you have reached Cape of Good Hope, where the mountain railroad rounded a point above Millard Canyon.

Over the next mile you pass the Dawn Mine Trail, leading left down into Millard Canyon (an option on your return trip if the area has been reopened to access; check with the US Forest Service), as well as the landmarks of Dawn Mine Station, Grand Circular Bridge, and Horseshoe Curve as the route climbs high along the east wall of Millard Canyon. Finally, the old roadbed turns east, passes through Granite Gate, ascends to near the head of Grand Canyon,

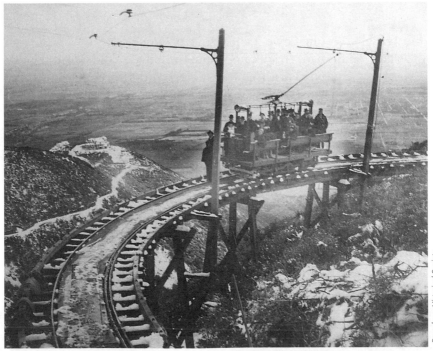

Pasadena Historical Society

The Grand Circular Bridge on the Mount Lowe Railway (1895)

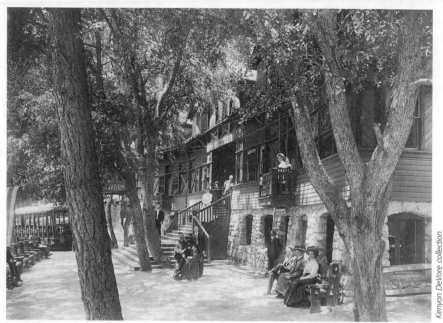

Ye Alpine Tavern, Mount Lowe Railway (circa 1914)

and reaches Mount Lowe Trail Camp on your left, 5.5 miles from the start. The shady trail camp—on the site of old Mount Lowe Tavern—is equipped with tables, stoves, and restrooms, but there is no good water here unless it is treated. You may wish to continue up the roadway, and then turn right at a junction, out to Inspiration Point, 0.5 mile from the campground. Here, on clear days, you are rewarded with a grand view down Castle Canyon to Echo Mountain and beyond over the lowlands to the distant sea.

Return the same way, or descend via Castle Canyon or the Upper Sam Merrill Trail to Echo Mountain (*see* Hike 23), and then go up the lower part of the railway bed to Sunset Ridge and return the way you came. Another option, closed as of this writing as part of the Station Fire Recovery Area, is to return the way you came, down the old roadbed, until you turn down the Dawn Mine Trail to Dawn Mine in Millard Canyon (*see* Hike 19). Any of these alternatives adds about 2 miles to the round-trip.

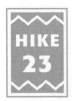

MOUNT LOWE RAILWAY LOOP TOUR

HIKE LENGTH: 12 miles round-trip; 2,800' elevation gain
DIFFICULTY: Moderate
SEASON: November–May
TOPO MAPS: *Pasadena, Mount Wilson*

Features

The old Mount Lowe Railway is long gone, remembered only by those who traveled in these mountains during the early decades of the 20th century. Yet it once attracted tourists by the thousands. No visit to Southern California was complete without taking the thrilling ride up the cable incline to Echo Mountain, and then the twisting trolley trip to rustic Ye Alpine Tavern, nestled deep in a forest cove on the slopes of Mount Lowe. When the mountain railway was built, it was considered one of the engineering wonders of the world.

The Mount Lowe Railway and resort complex was the idea of two visionary Pasadenans—Civil War balloonist and inventor Thaddeus S. C. Lowe and engineer David J. Macpherson. With Lowe supplying the capital and Macpherson directing operations, the railway was hacked out of the mountainside in three stages during 1892 to 1895. First was a trolley line from Altadena into Rubio Canyon, where the first of Lowe's popular edifices—Rubio Pavilion—was located (*see* Hike 25). Then an incline railway climbed 1,300 feet to Echo Mountain, where two hostelries—The Chalet and Echo Mountain House—were perched (*see* Hike 24). Finally, a 4-mile winding trolley ride, past airy viewpoints such as Horseshoe Curve, Cape of Good Hope, Grand Circular Bridge, and Granite Gate, carried awestruck visitors to Ye Alpine Tavern (later called Mount Lowe Tavern). Lowe was bankrupted by the venture, and for most of the 43 years of its operation, the Pacific Electric Railway Company ran the complex. From its opening in 1893 until the burning of Mount Lowe Tavern in 1936, the renowned mountain railway and resort complex was visited by an estimated 3 million persons.

Above Echo Mountain, the scars of the winding railway are clearly visible today, and it is possible to hike to the tavern site along its broken bed, the upper section of which is now part of the Sunset Ridge–Mount Lowe fire road (*see* Hike 22). At the old tavern site, under spreading oaks and big-cone Douglas-firs, the US Forest Service

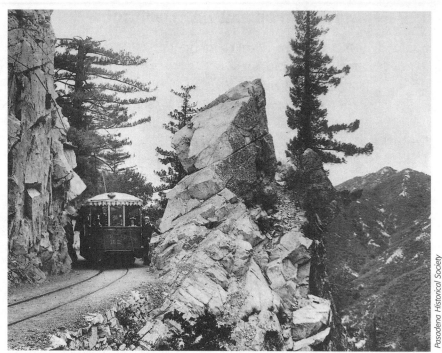

Pasadena Historical Society

The Granite Gate on the Mount Lowe Railway (circa 1915)

has constructed the Mount Lowe Trail Camp, with tables, stoves, restrooms, and a spring-fed drinking fountain. (As of this writing in spring 2013, the water is unsafe to drink—check with the US Forest Service for the latest status.)

A half mile out from the trail camp, overlooking the San Gabriel Valley, is the ramada at Inspiration Point, where tourists took in the view that was described in Mount Lowe Railway days as breathtaking, beautiful, and inspiring.

Over the years, much restoration work has been accomplished by weekend volunteers of the Scenic Mount Lowe Railway Historical Committee. Old trails have been cleared, artifacts have been uncovered and placed on display at Echo Mountain, and—their crowning achievement—the ramada at Inspiration Point was rebuilt and dedicated on November 16, 1996.

For those with vivid imaginations, it is possible to stand among the foundations of the mountain railway and picture oneself a part of Professor Lowe's dream come true. This loop trip is for those with such imaginations.

Description

Drive to the north end of Lake Avenue in Altadena and park alongside the road. To your right (east), near a large locked gate, is the beginning of the Sam Merrill Trail to Echo Mountain.

Follow the trail east, down across Las Flores Canyon, and up the slopes to Echo Mountain (*see* Hike 24). From Echo Mountain, turn north and follow the broad, graded railway bed around the head of Las Flores Canyon to Sunset Ridge, where you pick up the Sunset Ridge–Mount Lowe fire road. Turn right (north) and proceed up the fire road. You will begin to notice here the unmistakable scars of the 2009 Station Fire. Within the next mile, you pass such viewpoints of yesteryear as Cape of Good Hope, Horseshoe Curve, and most famous of all, Grand Circular Bridge. There is no bridge here now, just a sharp hairpin turn of the road. After following the slope above Millard Canyon for a mile, you round the mountain and turn east high above Grand Canyon, passing through the remains of the rock outcrop once known as Granite Gate. Four miles from Echo Mountain, you finally reach Mount Lowe Trail Camp, nestled in a grove of oaks and firs. The stone wall foundation just east of camp is all that remains of old Mount Lowe Tavern.

From the trail camp, continue up the fire road, going right (southeast) at a road junction, 0.5 mile to the ramada at Inspiration Point. Immediately east of the point is the marked trail dropping into Castle Canyon. Follow this narrow, 2-mile trail as it zigzags steeply down through fir- and oak-shaded Castle Canyon; around the head of Rubio Canyon, where you cross a small creek (which usually has water); and over to Echo Mountain again. Then descend the Sam Merrill Trail to Altadena.

An alternate route between Echo Mountain and Mount Lowe Trail Camp is the old Sunset Trail, signed at both ends as the SAM MERRILL TRAIL. From Echo Mountain, it starts up the crest of the ridge directly to the north; zigzags up and around what was known in Mount Lowe Railway days as Sunset Point; turns east, paralleling the old railway bed about 200 feet above it; and intersects the Mount Lowe fire road about 300 yards south of the trail camp. To locate the trail from above, follow the fire road 300 yards south from Mount Lowe Trail Camp to a road junction; the trail goes right (west) just south of the junction. This Sunset (or Upper Sam Merrill) Trail is regularly maintained by volunteers from Altadena and other nearby communities.

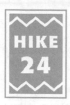

SAM MERRILL TRAIL:
ALTADENA TO ECHO MOUNTAIN

HIKE 24

HIKE LENGTH: 5 miles round-trip; 1,400' elevation gain
DIFFICULTY: Moderate
SEASON: November–May
TOPO MAPS: *Pasadena, Mount Wilson*

Features

If it were not for the efforts of a handful of public-spirited and sentimental Pasadena and Altadena residents, the Mount Lowe Railway would be all but forgotten today. These people have given freely of their time and effort in restorative projects, enabling today's visitor to relive some of this bygone era when cable cars and trolleys climbed high on the mountain.

One of these volunteer efforts was the construction and maintenance of the Sam Merrill Trail from Altadena to Echo Mountain. The trail was built during the 1930s by Charles Warner and the Forest Conservation Club of Pasadena to replace the original, overgrown footpath. During the 1940s it was maintained and improved by Samuel Merrill of Altadena, retired clerk of the Superior Court of Los Angeles. After Merrill's death in 1948, the pathway was named in his honor. Today this trail, one of the most popular in the San Gabriels, is kept in excellent condition by local volunteers.

Back in the early years of the Mount Lowe Railway, Echo Mountain was known as the White City. Perched on top were two hotels— Echo Mountain House and The Chalet—as well as a powerhouse, a machine shop, a dormitory, a reservoir, a small zoo, the Mount Lowe Observatory, and, so it would not be forgotten after dark, the world's most powerful searchlight. All but the searchlight were painted white, clearly visible from the valley below. To reach the White City, tourists were hoisted up the cable incline in white "chariots."

Through a series of fires and windstorms, the White City was destroyed—Echo Mountain House first (1900), then all but the observatory (1905), and finally the observatory itself (1928). The incline was abandoned in 1938.

Nothing but ruins remain today. To commemorate what once was here, a bronze plaque is embedded in cement next to the old incline bull wheel. Among the foundations, young Coulter pines and incense cedars, planted by conservation groups in 1941 and 1948, are growing tall.

This trip takes you up the Sam Merrill Trail to Echo Mountain, gives you a guided tour of where once stood the White City, and returns you the same way.

Description

Drive to the north end of Lake Avenue in Altadena and park alongside the road. To your right (east), near a large locked gate, is the beginning of the Sam Merrill Trail to Echo Mountain.

Follow the trail east alongside a fence; where it turns left (north), continue straight ahead and pick up the trail as it descends Las Flores Canyon and climbs up the east slope of the canyon. After 3 zigzagging miles, you reach the ridge behind (north of) Echo Mountain. Here, you intersect the old railway bed (*see* Hike 23). Turn right (south) and follow the railway bed about 100 yards to the Echo Mountain ruins. You come first to the commemorative plaque and the old incline bull wheel, embedded in cement. Just beyond, the wall on your left is the foundation of Echo Mountain House, and the pile of concrete rubble ahead is what remains of the incline depot and powerhouse, dynamited by the US Forest Service in 1959. From the steps of Echo Mountain House, you can look directly down the incline bed, descending 1,300 feet into Rubio Canyon. (Do not descend the incline; footing is loose and it is dangerous.) East of the Echo Mountain House site, 100 feet down the ridge, is the site of The Chalet. Nothing remains of this first hotel. The Mount Lowe Observatory, housing a 13-inch telescope, was located behind Echo Mountain, 0.25 mile up the ridge. Directly below the observatory was the reservoir.

After immersing yourself in history and taking in the view, return the way you came.

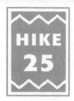

ALTADENA TO RUBIO CANYON

HIKE LENGTH: 1.5 miles round-trip; 200' elevation gain
DIFFICULTY: Easy
SEASON: November–May
TOPO MAP: *Mount Wilson*

Features

Rubio Canyon was once one of the premier scenic attractions of the San Gabriel Mountains, visited by thousands of tourists. For 43 years, 1893–1936, Rubio Canyon was an important way station on the Mount Lowe Railway. Tourists rode the winding electric trolley into the canyon, and then climbed aboard the white "chariots" for the ride up the cable incline to Echo Mountain. Professor Thaddeus S. C. Lowe's elegant Rubio Pavilion stood at the foot of the incline set amid a forest garden of sycamores, live oaks, ferns, and wildflowers. Radiating up and down the canyon from the edifice were more than a mile of planked walks and rustic stairways, leading through a picturesque setting of ferns, mossy nooks, and miniature waterfalls. All this came to an end in 1909, when a severe thunderstorm sent huge boulders crashing down upon the pavilion, demolishing the double-decked structure and causing the only death in all the years of the Mount Lowe operation. From then until the railway's end, Rubio Canyon was nothing but a transfer point for passengers bound for Mount Lowe Tavern.

Today this scene is difficult to visualize. Absolutely nothing remains of the magnificent pavilion that once spanned the canyon. The lower end of the incline has been completely eroded, and all the rails have been removed.

In 1998 workers hired by the Rubio Canyon Land and Water Association tried to reroute a water pipe damaged in the 1994 Northridge earthquake. While carving a notch in the steep canyonside, the workers accidentally triggered an avalanche that buried the little waterfalls and cascades under thousands of tons of boulders and debris.

The accident embarrassed the US Forest Service and outraged environmentalists, who demanded that the 100-foot-deep pile of rocks be removed. But federal officials denied responsibility for the cleanup, and the water company claimed that it didn't have the funds to pay for it. As a result, the landslide triggered a number of lawsuits and legal claims. However, a series of strong autumn storms in October

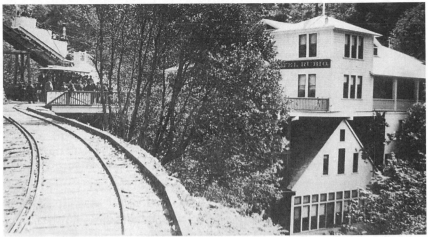

Kenyon DeVore collection

Rubio Pavilion (circa 1894)

2004 dumped more than 10 inches of rain on the area. In what must have been an awesome display, 50,000 tons of rock and debris had been swept away and strewn down the canyon. Old waterfalls were reborn and streams resumed their courses. Of course, there are still scars, and the area retains a raw, unkempt look that will take decades to soften, but it appears that Rubio Canyon is on the way to recovery.

Description

From Lake Avenue in Pasadena, drive north, past Altadena Drive, into Altadena. Turn right at Dolores Drive and follow it to Rubio Canyon Road. Follow it north to Rubio Crest Drive; turn left and then a quick right on Rubio Vista Drive. Park along the street. The trail begins on the east (right) side of the junction of Rubio Vista Drive and Pleasantridge Drive. Notice a narrow dirt path between the two houses on the corner, leading north into Rubio Canyon. Just beyond the houses lies the old railway bed that once took passengers to Rubio Pavilion.

Proceed along this eroded bed, mostly easygoing but overgrown in spots; near the end are two areas that may be troubling for very young hikers. In 0.5 mile you round a bend and run out of roadway; just beyond is the site of Rubio Pavilion. Carefully scramble down to the canyon bottom and pick your way among the boulders and debris up the canyon several hundred yards where a series of small waterfalls begins, the site of the old stairways and walkways. Return the way you came; it is not safe to continue farther unless you're an accomplished mountaineer.

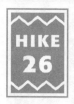

ALTADENA TO HENNINGER FLATS

HIKE LENGTH: 5.5 miles round-trip; 1,400' elevation gain
DIFFICULTY: Moderate
SEASON: November–June
TOPO MAP: *Mount Wilson*

Features

Above Altadena, the scars of the old Mount Wilson Toll Road are clearly visible, zigzagging sharply up the chaparral-covered mountainside from the mouth of Eaton Canyon. A rather conspicuous forested bench can be observed about a third of the way up. This is Henninger Flats (sometimes incorrectly spelled Henniger), home of the Los Angeles County Experimental Forestry Nursery.

The flats have a rich history. They were originally homesteaded by "Captain" William K. Henninger, who grew hay, corn, vegetables, fruit, and melons on his "farm in the clouds." In the early 1900s the flats were leased to the US Forest Service, and under the guidance of Theodore P. Lukens, the first scientific reforestation experiments in California were conducted. Thousands of seedlings from the nursery here were transplanted to fire-blackened slopes all over Southern California.

Since 1928 Henninger Flats and the surrounding slopes have been under the administration of Los Angeles County foresters. Under their care, thousands of new tree seedlings each year—knobcone pine, Coulter pine, Canary Island pine, Monterey pine, and Aleppo pine, as well as varieties of cypress, cedar, and sequoia—are grown. A new administration building with a museum on the ground floor, open to the public on weekends, displays reforestation and historical exhibits. A picnic area and public campground, set amid the shade of tall pines, are maintained by the county.

Be aware that the route is almost completely shadeless, and during warm weather the hike is best done early in the morning. Bring plenty of water; as of this writing—spring 2013—the water at the flats is unsafe to drink.

Description

Drive to the beginning of the old Mount Wilson Toll Road near the east loop of Pinecrest Drive in Altadena. Note that parking is restricted on Pinecrest Drive itself; you may need to park on one of the adjacent streets, being careful to comply with posted parking signs.

Walk past the locked gate, down across Eaton Canyon, and up the wide old road, zigzagging up steep chaparral-covered slopes just over 2.5 miles to Henninger Flats. Just inside the shady flats, on both sides of the road, are the picnic and campground. Straight ahead is the new administration building and museum. Behind the museum and to the right are the structures of the county reforestation nursery. A fire lookout tower, formerly atop Castro Peak in the Santa Monicas, stands as a historical exhibit to your left.

Return the same way you came. Do not try shortcuts down the chaparral-blanketed slopes.

Other options are to continue up the toll road to Mount Wilson (*see* Hike 27), or follow the Idlehour Trail into upper Eaton Canyon (*see* Hike 28).

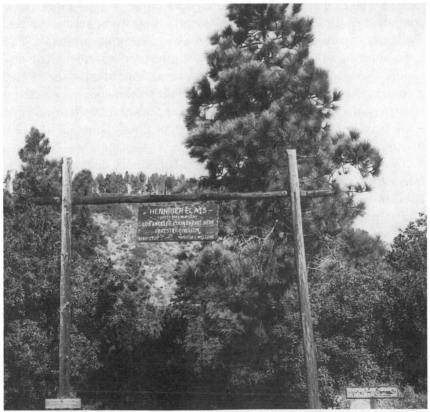

Henninger Flats, Los Angeles County Reforestation Nursery

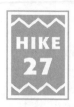

MOUNT WILSON TOLL ROAD

HIKE LENGTH: 9 miles one way;
4,500' elevation loss or gain
DIFFICULTY: Strenuous (uphill); moderate (downhill)
SEASON: November–June
TOPO MAP: *Mount Wilson*

Features

Back in the 1920s, when the age of the automobile arrived in Southern California, the Mount Wilson Toll Road was a favorite of strong-nerved drivers. Narrow, zigzagging, and cliff-hanging much of the way, without side rails, this auto route from Altadena to the summit of Mount Wilson often saw heavy holiday traffic. For those who preferred not to drive themselves, there was the popular Mount Wilson Stage, making the upward grind twice a day—more often when the traffic demanded. Surprisingly, there were few accidents. Evidently the obvious dangers served as a cautioning influence. The most amazing episode in the road's long history was the Altadena–Mount Wilson automobile race, held several times during the 1920s, a contest that makes the more famous Pikes Peak road race pale by comparison. The record for the 9-mile, 4,500-foot, 44-hairpin-turn event was 22 minutes flat, set by Pasadenan Frank Benedict in 1922, driving a Paige 6-66.

It was the Pasadena and Mount Wilson Toll Road Company, incorporated 1889, that first envisioned a road to the mountaintop. Two years later the company completed a 4-foot-wide toll trail to the summit—50 feet per rider, 25 feet per hiker. Not until 1907 was the trail widened to a 10-foot roadway, this to transport the 60-inch telescope to its mountaintop home. In 1912 the toll road was widened to 12 feet to accommodate the 100-inch telescope and was opened to the public, and for the next 24 years it was a popular Sunday drive except among the fainthearted. The end for this historic old route came in 1936. Superseded by the new Angeles Crest Highway, it was closed to the public and turned over to the US Forest Service for use as a fire road. So it remains today.

Mount Wilson, home of one of the world's great observatories, is probably the best-known mountain in Southern California. It was named for Benjamin Wilson, who built the first modern trail to its summit in 1864 (*see* Hike 39). The first telescope on the peak was the 13-inch refractor of the short-lived Harvard Observatory, 1889–1890. Since 1904, the famed Carnegie Observatory has been here, thanks to the enthusiasm and efforts of two farseeing men— astronomer George Ellery Hale and businessman-turned-philanthropist Andrew Carnegie. From its installation in 1917 until surpassed by the 200-incher on Palomar Mountain in 1946, the 100-inch Hooker reflector on Mount Wilson was the world's largest. Today the Mount Wilson observatory is operated on behalf of the Carnegie Institution by the nonprofit Mount Wilson Institute.

In 1948 television came to Mount Wilson in the form of transmitting stations for all seven Los Angeles channels. Mount Wilson's natural flora was supplemented by a man-made forest of antennae, towers, and domes, most of them visible from the valley below. Television not only came, but it also conquered. In 1964 Metromedia Inc., operators of Station KTTV, purchased the entire mountaintop from the old Mount Wilson Hotel Company. The rambling old hotel, a fixture on the mountain since 1915 (a previous hotel was built in 1905 and burned in 1913), was torn down, and in its place rose Skyline Park, complete with a pavilion, a children's zoo, and picnic areas. Metromedia deeded the mountaintop to the US Forest Service in 1976. Old-timers would hardly recognize the mountaintop today.

You can tackle the old toll road in two ways. The easier is to have someone drive you to Mount Wilson (19 miles from La Cañada), and then hike down. Much more strenuous is to hike up the road from Altadena. Either way, you are rewarded with a close-at-hand view of the abrupt, chaparral-coated south slope of the front range, and you will marvel at the fortitude and backbone of those who once drove this tortuous roadway to the sky. Bring plenty of water—the supply at Henninger Flats is, as of this writing in spring 2013, unfit to drink—and don't do it in warm weather, as much of the route traverses shadeless chaparral.

Description

To walk up the old toll road, drive to the lower entrance, guarded by a locked gate, near the east loop of Pinecrest Drive in Altadena. Parking in this area is quite restricted; you will need to park on one

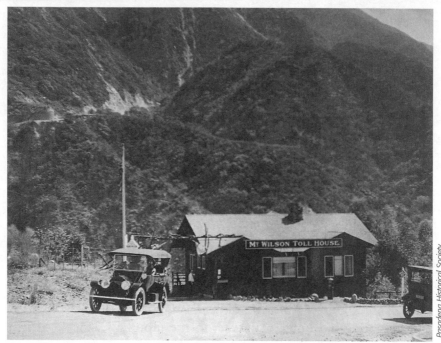

Pasadena Historical Society

Mt. Wilson Toll House (1914)

of the adjacent streets, being careful to note and comply with posted parking signs.

Proceed along the dirt roadway down across the mouth of Eaton Canyon and 2.75 miles up to Henninger Flats (*see* Hike 26). Continue on the road through the flats and up around a ridge. In another mile you pass the junction of the Idlehour Trail (*see* Hike 28), and just beyond, the site of George Schneider's old Halfway House, where perspiring travelers once enjoyed shade and refreshment. The toll road then zigzags up the ridge, rounds the south and east slopes of Mount Harvard, and reaches the Harvard-Wilson Saddle, site of old Martin's Camp, 8 miles from Altadena. After 1 more uphill mile you gain the Mount Wilson Circle Road just west of the entrance to Skyline Park. The entrance to the park, observatory grounds, museum, and café is through the gate immediately to the east of the loop road. It is open April 1–November 30. The café is currently open Friday–Sunday, 10 a.m.–5 p.m., during the months of April–November.

If you prefer to hike down the toll road, drive up the Angeles Crest Highway to Red Box, 14 miles from La Cañada, and then go right on the Mount Wilson Road to the loop road just outside the entrance to Skyline Park, 5 more miles. Immediately south of the entrance is the upper end of the old toll road, marked by a wooden sign.

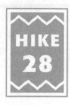

ALTADENA TO HENNINGER FLATS, IDLEHOUR TRAIL TO EATON CANYON, IDLEHOUR TRAIL CAMP, INSPIRATION POINT, CASTLE CANYON, ECHO MOUNTAIN

HIKE 28

HIKE LENGTH: 13 miles one way; 4,100' elevation gain
DIFFICULTY: Strenuous
SEASON: November–May
TOPO MAPS: *Mount Wilson, Pasadena*

Features

Few San Gabriel canyons compare with Eaton in ruggedness and inaccessibility. Precipitous sidewalls plunge down from lofty ridges to make this V-shaped gorge in the heart of the front range. A tumbling stream hurries down the length of the chasm, finally to plunge over idyllic Eaton Falls just above the canyon's mouth. The upper end of the canyon widens into a broad basin under the towering white faces of Mount Markham and San Gabriel Peak.

Trails into Eaton Canyon have always been difficult to build and maintain because of the rugged terrain. In decades past, you could hike directly up the canyon on a narrow footpath that clung to the side of the gorge above the stream, but the Pasadena Water Department fence has closed this approach. Today you avoid the difficult lower gorge by utilizing the Mount Wilson Toll Road to climb above the canyon, and then drop into its more gentle upper reaches via the Idlehour Trail.

You reach the canyon bottom at Idlehour Trail Camp, a secluded spot of unusual natural charm. Here, the creek experiences one of its few serene moods, and a fine forest of oaks, bays, and big-cone Douglas-firs provides cover. In this woodsy haunt once stood Camp Idle Hour, a small trail resort of the Great Hiking Era. The name signified the quiet, restful mood of the place, and throughout its existence (1915–1929), the camp was a favorite of lovers of sylvan seclusion.

The trip is a rather long one, involving much up and down, as all visits into upper Eaton Canyon must. But it samples some of the most scenic country in the front range—mostly untouched by the 2009 Station Fire. With a 2-mile car shuttle, your itinerary follows a great loop, dropping into Eaton Canyon from the east and climbing out via the west slope. If a car shuttle is not available, you can retrace your steps, covering just half of the loop. In any event, be in top shape; it's an all-day hike for most people.

Description

Leave one car at the Sam Merrill Trail entrance, at the head of Lake Avenue in Altadena. Drive the other to the beginning of the Mount Wilson Toll Road, near where Pinecrest Drive makes its east-end loop. Observe the posted signs carefully; parking is not as restricted on the adjacent streets.

Walk up the old toll road, passing Henninger Flats. One mile beyond the flats, where the toll road switchbacks up the slope to the right, look for the unsigned Idlehour Trail leading left, away from the toll road. Follow the trail over a slight rise and steeply down to Idlehour Trail Camp in Eaton Canyon. The camp, on a bench just east of the stream, is a good picnic or overnight spot, equipped with tables and stoves.

From Idlehour Trail Camp the trail goes upstream, passing the foundations of several old cabins. Much of the path here is washed out and you must boulder-hop. In 0.5 mile from the trail camp, look for the trail leaving the left side of the creek bed—it's easy to miss. Totaling 3 miles, the pathway turns sharply left (west), zigzags steeply up and around a ridge, contours into a side canyon (usually a small trickle of water), and continues up through an area burned by the 2009 Station Fire to meet a spur of the Mount Lowe fire road. Turn left (southeast) on the spur road to the cement foundation of old Inspiration Point, about 200 yards. Just east of the point is a signed trail dropping down Castle Canyon (*see* Hike 23). Follow this trail down to Echo Mountain, and then the Sam Merrill Trail (*see* Hike 24) to Lake Avenue in Altadena, 5 miles downhill all the way.

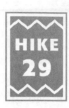

RED BOX TO SAN GABRIEL PEAK, MOUNT DISAPPOINTMENT

HIKE LENGTH: 6 miles round-trip; 1,500' elevation gain
DIFFICULTY: Moderate
SEASON: All year
TOPO MAPS: *Chilao Flat, Mount Wilson*

Features

Mount Disappointment (5,994') stands high on the crest of the front range, but not quite as high as its next-door summit, San Gabriel Peak. Hence the "disappointment" when some government surveyors lugged their equipment to the top in 1875, and then had to continue to the higher summit to do their surveying.

This trip follows the San Gabriel Peak Trail, built by the JPL Hiking Club in 1988; then the upper end of the Mount Disappointment fire road to gain the San Gabriel Peak–Mount Disappointment saddle; and then climbs both peaks. The views from both summits are panoramic. Sadly, the oak, fir, and pine forest that once shaded the upper reaches of both peaks was nearly all burned away in the 2009 Station Fire. It will take decades to grow back.

Description

Drive the 14 miles up Angeles Crest Highway from La Cañada to Red Box, and then turn right onto the Mount Wilson Road. Follow the latter about 0.33 mile to the beginning of the Mount Disappointment fire road on your right. Park here, but don't block the roadway. Be sure to display your Adventure Pass on your parked vehicle.

Take the San Gabriel Peak Trail, which begins about 50 feet to the left (east) of the fire-road gate. The trail switchbacks up, under a canopy of big-cone Douglas-firs and live oaks, to a junction with the upper section of the Mount Disappointment fire road, 1 mile. You begin to encounter evidence of the 2009 Station Fire that becomes more widespread as you near the top. Proceed 200 yards up the fire road to the ridgetop. Take the trail left, which drops 50 feet to the San Gabriel Peak–Mount Disappointment saddle and then climbs the west ridge of San Gabriel Peak to the summit, 0.5 mile.

On your return, follow the fire road through the charred remains of the forest that once grew here to the summit of Mount Disappointment, 0.25 mile from the saddle. The top is cluttered with

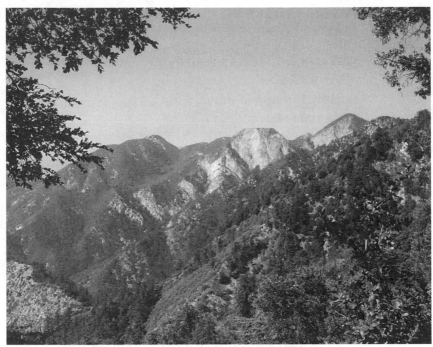

Mount Lowe, Mount Markham, and San Gabriel Peak

electronic installations and empty buildings dating from the 1950s, when an Army Nike missile station was located here.

Descend the way you came or take the fire road all the way down. Either route leads back to your car, but the fire road is a mile longer.

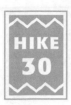

EATON SADDLE TO MARKHAM SADDLE, MOUNT LOWE

HIKE 30

HIKE LENGTH: 3 miles round-trip; 500' elevation gain
DIFFICULTY: Easy
SEASON: November–June
TOPO MAP: *Mount Wilson*

Features

This is the easy way to do historic Mount Lowe. You start from the back side—the Mount Wilson Road—and contour across the white diorite cliffs of San Gabriel Peak to Markham Saddle. Then climb the gentle north slope of the mountain through fire-thinned chaparral and clusters of small oak trees to the bare summit.

In the early days it was called Oak Mountain, for the groves of splendid live oaks on its upper slopes. By this name it was known when Professor Thaddeus S. C. Lowe and a party of leading Pasadena residents ascended it on horseback in 1892. Lowe was showing his friends his proposed mountain railway, then just beginning construction. One of the party proposed the name Mount Lowe in honor of the man in their midst. The motion was carried by a chorus of ayes, and in the words of publicist and writer G. Wharton James, "There above the clouds, it was named; and it will continue to be so named when every one of the party present at the christening shall have been laid away in Mother Earth; and generations yet unborn shall trace its rugged outlines on their physical geographies and call it Mount Lowe."

Lowe planned to continue his mountain railway to the top and construct a summit hotel, but he ran out of funds after reaching the site of Ye Alpine Tavern 1,000 feet below. During the years of the Mount Lowe Railway, untold thousands climbed to the top via two well-graded trails from the tavern. On the summit were a small, open observation pavilion and a series of view tubes (iron pipes) pointed at various attractions below.

With the burning of Mount Lowe Tavern in 1936 and the abandoning of the mountain railway, visits to Mount Lowe almost ceased, and the trails and summit paraphernalia fell into decay. Thankfully, Sierra Club volunteers have restored one of the trails, polished and relettered the old view tubes, and left a new register book with pictures of the Mount Lowe of old. Old Mount Lowe is again worth visiting.

Description

Drive up the Angeles Crest Highway 14 miles from La Cañada to Red Box. Turn right on the Mount Wilson Road 2.5 miles to Eaton Saddle. The saddle is unnamed on maps but easy to locate: it is the first spot past Red Box where the highway touches the top of the ridge and you can look south. Be sure to display your Adventure Pass on your parked vehicle.

Walk past the locked gate onto the Mount Lowe fire road, overlooking the yawning chasm of upper Eaton Canyon. Follow the road as it turns west and contours around the precipitous south face of San Gabriel Peak. Near midpoint, the road tunnels through a nearly vertical cliff. Notice the old guardrails outside the wall, remnants of the airy old Cliff Trail that once joined Mount Lowe Tavern with Mount Wilson. After a short mile you reach Markham Saddle, a V-shaped cleft between San Gabriel Peak and Mount Markham. Here, you leave the road and take an unmarked footpath to the left that leads southwest around the slopes of Mount Markham to the saddle between Mount Markham and Mount Lowe. You then enter a forest of small oaks as the trail rounds the east slope of Mount Lowe. About 300 yards beyond this last saddle, look for an unmarked side trail branching back to your right (west). Leave the main trail (which continues down to Mount Lowe Trail Camp) and walk up the side footpath about 0.25 mile to the bare summit of Mount Lowe.

After enjoying the fine vista over the front-range country and pondering the history of this place, return the way you came.

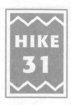

EATON SADDLE TO MOUNT LOWE TRAIL CAMP, MOUNT LOWE FIRE ROAD

HIKE LENGTH: 6 miles round-trip;
700' elevation gain and loss
DIFFICULTY: Moderate
SEASON: November–June
TOPO MAP: *Mount Wilson*

Features

This loop trip takes you completely around Mount Lowe and visits secluded Mount Lowe Trail Camp, once the location of famed Mount Lowe Tavern (*see* Hike 23). Most of the hike is via easy-graded fire road, but about 2 miles are on the historic, oak-shaded Mount Lowe "East" Trail, recently reworked into good condition. You are rewarded en route with superb vistas down into Eaton Canyon and fire-ravaged Bear and Grand Canyons and, if the atmosphere is clear, down the south slope of the front range to the sprawling San Gabriel Valley.

Description

Drive up the Angeles Crest Highway 14 miles from La Cañada to Red Box. Turn right on the Mount Wilson Road 2.5 miles to Eaton Saddle. Be sure to display your Adventure Pass on your parked vehicle.

Walk past the locked gate and follow the Mount Lowe fire road to Markham Saddle, and then turn left on the Mount Lowe "East" Trail to the saddle between Mounts Markham and Lowe (*see* Hike 30 for details). Continue on the trail through a shady oak forest around the east shoulder of Mount Lowe, and then down around the south slope via switchbacks to a badly eroded firebreak. The trail crosses the firebreak and continues zigzagging down to the Mount Lowe fire road. Follow it south 100 yards to a junction with the Inspiration Point spur road, and then right about 300 yards to Mount Lowe Trail Camp. Here, under oaks and firs, there are tables, stoves, restrooms, and a spring-fed drinking fountain (the water is unsafe to drink as of this writing in spring 2013). The stone foundation adjacent to the camp is all that remains of old Mount Lowe Tavern, once the scene of much merrymaking.

To return, retrace your steps up the fire road to the Inspiration Point junction. Go left and follow the road northwest around Mount

Lowe's long west ridge, and then east back across Markham Saddle and San Gabriel Peak's white cliffs to Eaton Saddle.

An option is to return via the Old Mount Lowe "West" Trail, overgrown and thorny but passable—wear long pants. You will be delighted to come across several of the old view tubes—iron pipes aimed at landmarks below—placed along the trail years ago. About 300 yards up the Mount Lowe fire road from the Inspiration Point spur road—almost directly north of and above Mount Lowe Trail Camp—the trail zigzags up the west slope of a ravine, and then contours around the hillside to your left, paralleling the fire road about 200 feet above it. (The trail you see climbing to the right connects with the Mount Lowe "East" Trail.) You contour and climb westward 0.5 mile, passing several of the old view tubes, and then round the ridge and ascend steadily east, with two switchbacks near the top, to Mount Lowe's bare summit. From the summit, descend the beaten path back to the Mount Lowe "East" Trail (*see* Hike 30), and then walk left to Markham Saddle and via the fire road back to Eaton Saddle.

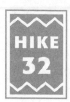

EATON SADDLE TO MARKHAM SADDLE, SAN GABRIEL PEAK

HIKE LENGTH: 3.5 miles round-trip; 1,000' elevation gain
DIFFICULTY: Moderate
SEASON: November–June
TOPO MAP: *Mount Wilson*

Features

Pyramidal San Gabriel Peak towers high on the crest of the front range. From its 6,161-foot summit, you get an unmatched 360-degree panorama over the wrinkled San Gabriel Mountains, with the front range in the foreground, laced as it is with paved highways, fire roads, trails, firebreaks, and assorted paraphernalia of mankind. Your vista is good because the top is tall, small, and apical. As on nearby Strawberry Peak (*see* Hike 36), you get that airy, top-of-the-world feeling.

There are days—increasing in number—when you look down upon canyon-ascending arms of smog, rising from the vast megalopolis dimly visible to the south. There are other days when billowing clouds swirl around you, playing hide-and-seek with nearby peaks. And there are those rare winter and spring days when the sky has been washed clean by a storm, and you can see half of Southern California spread out in stark beauty. These are the days to climb San Gabriel Peak.

This climb is short in distance, but the trail is steep and narrow in spots, so wear lug-soled boots.

Description

Drive up the Angeles Crest Highway 14 miles from La Cañada to Red Box. Turn right up the Mount Wilson Road to Eaton Saddle, 2.5 miles. The saddle is unmarked on maps but easy to locate: it is the first spot after Red Box where the highway touches a gap in the ridge and you can look south. Be sure to display your Adventure Pass on your parked vehicle.

Walk past the locked gate and across the rugged south face of San Gabriel Peak via the Mount Lowe fire road 0.5 mile to Markham Saddle. At the saddle, just beyond the water tank, turn sharply right (north) and pick up a brushy, unmarked trail leading up the mountainside. Follow the trail up one switchback, and then across the west slope of San Gabriel Peak to the high saddle between Mount

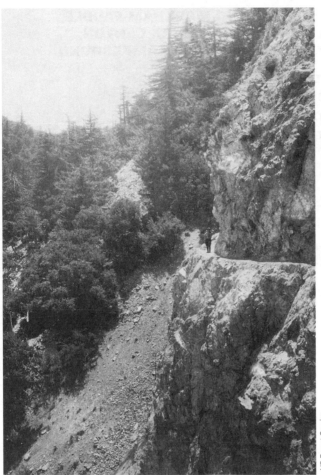

US Forest Service

**Famous Cliff Trail between Eaton Saddle and
Markham Saddle, now bypassed by Mueller Tunnel**

Disappointment and San Gabriel Peak, about 0.75 mile. Part of this
pathway is eroded where it crosses the steep slope, so watch your
step. At the saddle, turn right (east) and follow a steep climbers' trail
up the ridge to the top.

After enjoying your eagle's-eye view, return the way you came.
Do not try to descend directly down the ridge (southeast) to Eaton
Saddle—the footing is unstable and the chaparral is thick and thorny.

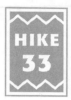

EATON SADDLE TO MARKHAM SADDLE, TOM SLOAN SADDLE, BEAR CANYON, ARROYO SECO, SWITZER CAMPGROUND

HIKE LENGTH: 10 miles one way;
2,500' elevation loss, 700' elevation gain
DIFFICULTY: Moderate
SEASON: November–June
TOPO MAPS: *Mount Wilson, Pasadena, Condor Peak*

Features

This trip is a long walk through some of the most scenic parts of the front-range country. The first 8 miles are all downhill, and the last 2 miles are uphill. One may especially enjoy the descent of Bear Canyon—recovering slowly from the 2009 Station Fire—to the middle gorge of the Arroyo Seco via the remnant of the old Tom Sloan Trail, a historic footpath that once joined two of the most popular resorts in the mountains—Mount Lowe Tavern and Switzer's. With the demise of the tavern in 1936, the trail fell into disuse, and now much of it is overgrown. However, the stretch through Bear Canyon remains passable, although partly washed out. A car shuttle between Eaton Saddle and Switzer's Picnic Area, 6 miles apart on the Angeles Crest Highway, is required.

Description

Drive up the Angeles Crest Highway 10.5 miles from La Cañada to the side road down to Switzer's Picnic Area, 0.5 mile past the junction of the Angeles Crest and Angeles Forest Highways. Turn right and descend 0.25 mile to the parking area outside the picnic area. Leave one car here. Drive the other 4 miles up the Angeles Crest to Red Box, and then go right 2.5 miles on the Mount Wilson Road to Eaton Saddle. Be sure to display your Adventure Pass on your parked vehicle.

Walk past the locked gate, following the Mount Lowe fire road across the face of San Gabriel Peak to Markham Saddle, and then on down the road until it reaches the top of Mount Lowe's long west ridge, 1.75 miles from the start. Here, the road switches back eastward. Leave the road here and proceed down the obvious but unmarked trail on the right (north) side of the ridge to Tom Sloan Saddle, a brushy 0.75 mile. From the saddle, follow the old Tom

Sloan Trail as it drops northwest down into Bear Canyon. You reach the canyon floor in 0.5 mile, a beautiful spot shaded by big-cone Douglas-firs. The impact of the fire is much less here, and the canyon has retained its woodsy charm.

The foundations you see are all that remain of several old cabins, abandoned after a fire many years ago. Continue down Bear Canyon, following the streamside trail, or boulder-hopping where the trail has been washed out, to Bear Canyon Trail Camp, located on a shaded bench on the south side of the creek, about 2 miles from Tom Sloan Saddle. Here is a perfect lunch stop, as it lies about halfway on your trip.

After lunch, continue down-canyon, partly on trail, partly boulder-hopping, to the junction with the Arroyo Seco, 2 more miles. Turn right (north) up the Arroyo Seco and follow the trail past the delightful pools and cascades of the middle gorge to a difficult-to-spot junction where the trail climbs out of the canyon to the main Arroyo Seco Trail above Switzer Falls (*see* Hike 17 for details). If you reach the foot of Switzer Falls, you've gone 0.25 mile too far up the canyon. (Under no circumstances should you try to climb over the falls.) When you reach the main Arroyo Seco Trail high on the ridge, turn right (north) and follow the well-beaten footpath through Commodore Switzer Trail Camp and on to Switzer's Picnic Area (*see* Hike 17).

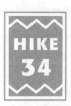

SIERRA MADRE TO BAILEY CANYON, JONES PEAK

HIKE LENGTH: 7 miles round-trip; 2,300' elevation gain
DIFFICULTY: Moderate
SEASON: November–May
TOPO MAP: *Mount Wilson*

Features

Towering directly over the small foothill community of Sierra Madre, 3,375-foot Jones Peak divides the watersheds of the Little Santa Anita Canyon (*see* Hikes 39 and 40) to the east, and rugged, steep, narrow Bailey Canyon, where this trip originates.

The canyon was homesteaded in 1875 by R. J. Bailey, but he soon sold it and the property passed through a succession of titleholders. Today it is owned by the city of Sierra Madre, which operates it as Bailey Canyon Park. Jones Peak was named for the first mayor of Sierra Madre, C. W. Jones, who served 1907–1914 and was a long-time resident of the town, living to the ripe old age of 99 before his death in 1967.

Most of the trail is shadeless and, if the day is sunny, hot. Do it early in the morning or on a cool winter or spring day, and wear sturdy boots for the final, steep scramble to the peak.

Description

In Sierra Madre, take Baldwin Avenue north from the 210 freeway, to its end at Carter Avenue; turn left and proceed 0.5 mile to the parking lot for Bailey Canyon Park. The park is open sunrise–sunset, so plan accordingly.

From the northwest corner of the parking lot, head west past the picnic area and exit through a turnstile onto a paved road. Head north, toward the canyon, clearly visible ahead. The road soon turns to dirt and becomes a footpath, and you reach a junction. Bear right as the trail begins to head uphill. The trail switchbacks steeply up the east wall of the canyon, and in just over 2 miles you enter the welcome shade of a live oak forest near the ruins of a small cabin, a nice spot for a break. Continue up the trail as it climbs another 700 feet to a saddle just north of the peak. From here, it's a short but steep scramble up to the top. If it's a clear day, you are rewarded with a spectacular vista of the San Gabriel Valley, downtown Los Angeles,

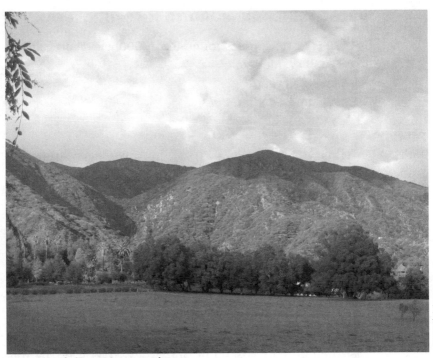

Jones Peak from Sierra Madre

and, if it's exceptionally clear, Catalina. Below, to the east, you look down on the Mount Wilson Trail and Little Santa Anita Canyon.

Return the way you came, taking care to watch your footing on the descent. One very scenic and interesting option is to take the faint use trail that continues from the saddle north up the ridge a short distance to where the ridge veers left. Look for a crude sign denoting a trail branching off to the right that quickly begins to descend steeply into Little Santa Anita Canyon, reaching the bottom in a short mile. The trail dumps you out in a small streambed that quickly intersects the Mount Wilson Trail. Turn right here and hike downhill past First Water and back to Mira Monte Avenue in Sierra Madre, another 3 miles. This option requires a short car shuttle, or you can hike on surface streets back to your car, just under a mile, for a total trip distance of 8 miles.

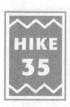

JOSEPHINE FIRE ROAD TO JOSEPHINE PEAK

HIKE 35

HIKE LENGTH: 8 miles round-trip; 1,900' elevation gain
DIFFICULTY: Moderate
SEASON: All year
TOPO MAP: *Condor Peak*

Features

Note: As of this writing, spring 2013, this hike lies within the Station Fire Recovery Area and is closed to entry. Check with the US Forest Service to verify the current status of this area before attempting this hike.

Josephine Peak—at 5,558 feet, the high point of the prominent spur extending 2 miles west from Strawberry Peak—offers superb views of the Big Tujunga watershed. A well-graded fire road climbs 4 miles from the Angeles Forest Highway to the fire lookout on the summit. This makes for a pleasant stroll when the weather is mild. Don't try it on a hot day; except for a few forested spots near the top, the route is devoid of shade. An option, if you are in top physical condition, is to climb both Josephine and Strawberry Peaks by this approach, descending either the same way or via Colby Canyon (*see* Hike 36).

The origin of the name Josephine is obscure. As early as 1889 there was a Josephine Gold Mine in the upper Big Tujunga. Several authorities believe that the peak was named for the wife of J. B. Lippencott, a U.S. Geological Survey employee who used the summit as a triangulation point while mapping the mountains in 1894. Another source claims that it was named for the daughter of Phil Begue, one of the early forest rangers in the range. The fire lookout, erected in 1937, burned down in the 1976 Big Tujunga fire.

Description

From La Cañada, drive up the Angeles Crest Highway 10 miles to the junction with the Angeles Forest Highway, opposite the Clear Creek Ranger Station. Park off the highway alongside the ranger station. Be sure to display your Adventure Pass on your parked vehicle.

The Josephine fire road begins on the east side of the Angeles Forest Highway about 50 yards north of the junction. Walk past the locked gate up the road. The 2-mile route climbs the ridge dividing Colby Canyon from Clear Creek and zigzags to the crest of Josephine's east

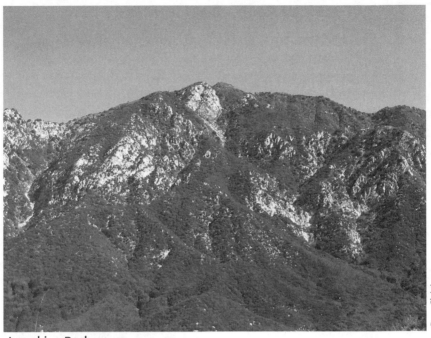

Doug Christiansen

Josephine Peak

ridge. Here, the junction goes right (east) to Josephine Saddle and Strawberry Peak (*see* Hike 36) and left (west) to Josephine Peak. Go left, following the road through oaks and firs on the north side of the ridge to the concrete foundation of the summit lookout.

Return by the same route, or if you can arrange a 1-mile car shuttle, descend to Josephine Saddle and down the old Colby Canyon Trail to the Angeles Crest Highway (*see* Hike 36). Don't take trailless short-cuts that may look tempting; the chaparral is thick and thorny.

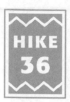

COLBY CANYON TO STRAWBERRY PEAK

HIKE LENGTH: 6 miles round-trip; 2,600' elevation gain
DIFFICULTY: Moderate
SEASON: All year
TOPO MAPS: *Condor Peak, Chilao Flat*

Features

Note: As of this writing, spring 2013, this hike lies within the Station Fire Recovery Area and is closed to entry. Check with the US Forest Service to verify the current status of this area before attempting this hike.

Strawberry Peak, a lump-shaped mass of granite boulders rising 6,164 feet above sea level, is the highest of all the summits of the San Gabriel front range. Looming far above the Angeles Crest Highway between the Arroyo Seco and Big Tujunga watersheds, its airy crown commands a sweeping vista over mountain and lowland.

Strawberry is the only peak in the front range whose ascent involves more than a plodding walk up. Its nearly vertical upper ramparts give you a taste of the alpinist's exhilaration, and once on top you'll really know that you've climbed a mountain. There, with slopes tapering precipitously on all sides, you get that top-of-the-world feeling. Many hikers consider it the "fun" peak of the San Gabriels.

The peak was labeled by wags at Switzer's Camp back in the 1880s, who fancied a resemblance to a strawberry standing on its stem. It has been a popular climb as long as modern man has trod the San Gabriels. During the Great Hiking Era (1895–1938), backpackers chugging over the well-beaten trail between Switzer's and Colby's often made the airy side trip to take in the rewarding summit panorama. It is just as frequented today. Every fair-weather weekend finds climbers by the scores testing their stamina and skills on its steep granite spine.

The climb is not particularly difficult for those in good physical condition who have had some experience on class 3 rock. Using proper caution—testing hand- and footholds and moving slowly—you should have little trouble if you follow the route indicated by green arrows painted at intervals on boulders. Lug-soled boots are strongly recommended. Extra care should be taken on the descent, for that is when most accidents occur.

Description

Drive up the Angeles Crest Highway to the Colby Canyon parking area, 11 miles from La Cañada and 1 mile beyond the junction of the Angeles Crest and Angeles Forest Highways. Be sure to display your Adventure Pass on your parked vehicle.

Proceed up the Colby Canyon Trail, which starts on the left (west) side of the creek. This trail is one of the historic pathways of the range. It is passable, although eroded in some spots and brushy in others. The trail follows the creek for 0.25 mile, and then climbs steeply up the right side to bypass several small waterfalls where the canyon narrows. You then drop back into the shady, alder-filled upper canyon before switchbacking up through thorny chaparral to Josephine Saddle, 2 miles from the highway. Here, you meet the Strawberry Spur of the Josephine fire road. An alternate way to reach this saddle—0.5 mile longer but easier going—is to follow the fire road from Clear Creek Ranger Station (*see* Hike 35).

From Josephine Saddle, the old Colby Canyon Trail winds eastward, around the north flank of Strawberry Peak and down to Strawberry Meadow (*see* Hike 38). Do *not* take this trail; instead climb eastward up a steep climbers' path that ascends the crest of the ridge. About 0.25 mile above Josephine Saddle you must negotiate a rocky section of about 75 vertical feet before continuing along the ridge crest 0.75 mile to the base of Strawberry Peak's imposing granite summit block. Here, the fainthearted will turn back; the route looks more difficult than it actually is and has some exposure. Follow the faded green arrows painted at intervals on the rock face, gripping firmly and testing hand- and footholds, to the final summit ridge, and then scramble a hundred feet to the top.

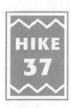

RED BOX TO STRAWBERRY PEAK, JOSEPHINE SADDLE, COLBY CANYON

HIKE 37

HIKE LENGTH: 7 miles round-trip; 1,500' elevation gain
DIFFICULTY: Moderate
SEASON: All year
TOPO MAPS: *Chilao Flat, Condor Peak*

Features

Note: As of this writing, spring 2013, this hike lies within the Station Fire Recovery Area and is closed to entry. Check with the US Forest Service to verify the current status of this area before attempting this hike.

This trip climbs Strawberry Peak by the east slope—the easy way—and then continues down the precipitous west face to Josephine Saddle and Colby Canyon via the standard route (*see* Hike 36). If you are unfamiliar with third-class rock scrambling, don't do the whole traverse—return from the peak to Red Box, the same way you came. For the entire traverse here described, a car shuttle between Red Box and Colby Canyon—4 miles apart on the Angeles Crest Highway—is required. The hike and the peak scramble, staying high on the ridge most of the way, offer panoramic vistas over the front range and the Upper Big Tujunga–Alder Creek backcountry. Wear lug-soled boots; much of the peak climb and descent is an off-trail scramble over granite boulders.

Description

Drive up the Angeles Crest Highway to Colby Canyon, 11 miles from La Cañada and 1 mile beyond the Clear Creek junction. Leave one car here and drive the other vehicle to Red Box Ranger Station, 4 miles farther up the highway. Be sure to display your Adventure Pass on your parked vehicles.

Cross the Angeles Crest Highway and follow it northeast about 50 yards to the beginning of the Barley Flats fire road. Turn left (north) and proceed up the fire road. In 0.5 mile you will come to a trail leading up to the left. Follow this path up to the ridge just south of Mount Lawlor, and then pick up an obvious but unmarked trail that contours around the mountain, high above the Angeles Crest Highway, to the saddle between Lawlor and Strawberry Peak—2 miles from the start. From the saddle, turn left (northwest) and follow a faint

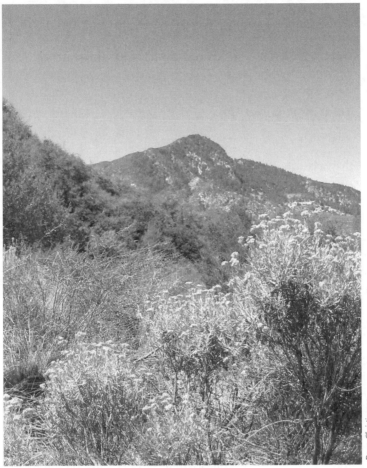

Doug Christiansen

Strawberry Peak

climbers' pathway up the ridge, through chaparral and over boulders, to the summit—an 800-foot gain in 0.75 mile.

Descend the abrupt west face, following the green arrows painted on the rocks, and then continue down the ridge to Josephine Saddle and descend Colby Canyon to the Angeles Crest Highway (*see* Hike 36 for route description). If you don't like the west face's steep rock descent, return to Red Box the way you came.

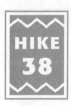

RED BOX TO STRAWBERRY SPRING, STRAWBERRY MEADOW

HIKE LENGTH: 8 miles round-trip; 1,400' elevation gain
DIFFICULTY: Moderate
SEASON: All year
TOPO MAP: *Chilao Flat*

Features

Note: As of this writing, spring 2013, this hike lies within the Station Fire Recovery Area and is closed to entry to allow the forest to recover. Check with the US Forest Service to verify the current status of this trail before attempting this hike.

The back side of Strawberry Peak holds pleasant surprises. Close under granite cliffs and boulder-stacked ridges, springs seep cold water and little meadows sprout tall grasses. In the protective shade of the great mountain, forest and chaparral intermingle and grow lush and green. Here, just across the ridge from the busy Angeles Crest Highway, away from ranger stations, public campgrounds, and the assorted miscellany that accompanies civilization, you savor a small touch of wilderness.

This delightful trail trip takes you over the mountain from Red Box to Strawberry Meadow—three small meadows below the great north cliff of Strawberry Peak. You pass alternately through clusters of dense chaparral—scrub oaks, manzanitas, snowbrushes, and mountain mahoganies—and a varied forest of live oaks, big-cone Douglas-firs, and Jeffrey and Coulter pines. The footpath that winds through this wilderness garden is old and little-traveled, making it all the more appealing. Bring lunch and a good book—you'll want to stay awhile.

Description

Drive up the Angeles Crest Highway to Red Box Ranger Station, 14 miles above La Cañada. Be sure to display your Adventure Pass on your parked vehicle.

Cross the Angeles Crest Highway and follow it northeast about 50 yards to the beginning of the Barley Flats fire road. Follow the road 0.5 mile, and then turn left and follow the trail up to the ridge and around the mountain to the saddle between Mount Lawlor and Strawberry Peak (*see* Hike 37).

From the saddle, continue on the trail as it gently descends around the east and northeast slopes of Strawberry Peak. The first 0.25 mile is in fine shape; beyond, the path is narrow and eroded in spots but not difficult to follow. You pass through alternate stretches of chaparral on sun-exposed slopes and forest on shady north faces. About 1 mile from the saddle you enter a woodsy recess and reach Strawberry Spring, flowing icy cold in spring and early summer. Then you cross a ridge and get your first glimpse of the lower meadow of Strawberry Meadow, with the great north cliff as an imposing backdrop. The trail drops steeply into a forested gully below the meadow and continues over another low ridge and down to Colby Ranch, a retreat for young Methodists. You won't go that far.

Just beyond the low point where the trail crosses the forested gully, look for a side trail marked with red-paint arrows on rocks leading back to the left (southwest). Turn sharply left and follow this footpath to the lower meadow of Strawberry Meadow, about 0.25 mile. You can stop here and enjoy the grassy clearing surrounded by oaks, pines, and boulder ridges, or you can continue up the red-marked trail another 0.5 mile, past a second small meadow, to the westernmost and largest clearing, right beneath the towering granite cliffs. Here, under magnificent Coulter pines, are two picnic tables placed by young Methodists from Colby Ranch.

After you've fully savored this delightful sanctuary, you have three options. The easiest is to return to Red Box the way you came. Or you can continue on down to Colby Ranch, if you have arranged a car shuttle and have permission from the operators of this private retreat. Or—if you can arrange a car shuttle—you can take the recently rebuilt Colby Canyon Trail, which leaves Strawberry Meadow near its upper (southwest) edge and climbs westward, and then contours the north slope around to Josephine Saddle, 2 miles. From here, you can descend the Colby Canyon Trail to the Angeles Crest Highway (*see* Hike 36).

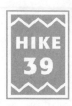

SIERRA MADRE TO ORCHARD CAMP

HIKE LENGTH: 7 miles round-trip; 2,000' elevation gain
DIFFICULTY: Moderate
SEASON: November–May
TOPO MAP: *Mount Wilson*

Features

Beautiful Little Santa Anita Canyon is steeped in history. Ages before the arrival of the white man, Gabrielino Indians forged a rough footpath up the canyon and on to Mount Wilson. Its namesake, Benjamin Wilson—proprietor of the Lake Vineyard Rancho in what is now San Marino, and a prominent Southern California resident—built the first modern trail into the San Gabriels up this canyon in 1864 to obtain timber from the mountaintop. In 1889 the Harvard University telescope was toted up this trail piece by piece, on its way to occupy the first observatory on Mount Wilson.

In a secluded glen, shaded by giant canyon oaks and big-cone Douglas-firs near the head of the main canyon, Don Benito—as Wilson was known to his many California friends—built his Halfway House in 1864. This original Halfway House, so named because it was midway between Sierra Madre and Mount Wilson, was a construction camp for the original Mount Wilson Trail. Later it was homesteaded by two colorful mountaineers, George Aiken and George Islip, who planted a small grove of apple, cherry, plum, and chestnut trees. With the maturing of these trees, the place became known as Orchard Camp. Around 1890 James McNally made Orchard Camp into a trail resort, and for 50 years this hostelry, under a succession of owners, was one of the most popular in the range. Its peak year was 1911, when more than 40,000 persons signed the camp register. Orchard Camp was abandoned in 1940. Today the buildings and tents are gone. But the enchanting streamside spot still holds appeal for lovers of sylvan seclusion.

Today most of Little Santa Anita Canyon lies within the Sierra Madre Historical Wilderness Area, owned by the city of Sierra Madre. For years, Ambrose Zaro, "the grand old man" of the trail, almost single-handedly maintained it. His death in March 1990 was mourned by all Mount Wilson Trail hikers.

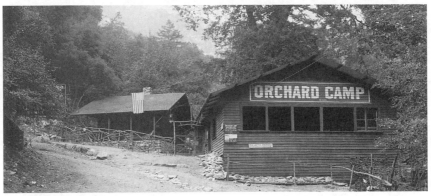

Orchard Camp (circa 1915)

Our very pleasant trail trip follows this historic footpath from Sierra Madre to old Orchard Camp and back. Take along a picnic lunch and a camera; you'll be so delighted by the woodsy charm of Orchard Camp that you'll want to stay awhile.

Description

Drive to the junction of Mira Monte Avenue and Mount Wilson Trail Drive in Sierra Madre. Do not leave your car above the immediate area of the junction; Mount Wilson Trail Drive is a private road.

Proceed about 150 yards up Mount Wilson Trail Drive to the beginning of the Mount Wilson Trail, marked by a large wooden sign on the left. Follow the trail alongside some private homes up to the ridgetop road, where the main footpath begins. Proceed up the trail as it climbs steadily along the west slope of the canyon, far above the stream. In 1.5 miles you reach a junction. The main trail goes straight ahead, staying high above the stream, climbing steadily. The trail branching right drops to the creek, the site of old Quarterway House, and meanders along the alder-shaded stream for a short distance. From the junction, continue on the main trail as it makes its way up the canyon until you round a ridge and enter the welcome shade of a live oak forest. The trail climbs steadily for another mile, and then drops to the small creek trickling down from Decker Spring. Beyond, you climb steeply, and then contour 0.5 mile through cool forest to Orchard Camp, located on an oak- and fir-shaded bench just above the sparkling creek. The huge canyon oak tree here is one of the oldest and largest oaks in the range. (A core test places its age at 1,500 years.)

Return the way you came.

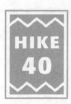

OLD MOUNT WILSON TRAIL

HIKE 40

HIKE LENGTH: 7 miles one way; 4,500' elevation gain
DIFFICULTY: Strenuous (uphill); moderate (downhill)
SEASON: November–May
TOPO MAP: *Mount Wilson*

Features

This original trail up Mount Wilson—forged by Benjamin Wilson in 1864—has, over the years, been one of the premier attractions in the range. No trail in the range has a richer heritage. (Its early history, an integral part of the Little Santa Anita Canyon story, is told in Hike 39.) During the Great Hiking Era (1895–1938), the dusty pathway vibrated under the tramp of boots and the pounding of hooves every fair-weather weekend. Every Saturday morning, hundreds would disembark from the red Pacific Electric trolley cars in Sierra Madre, knapsacks slung over their shoulders, and ramble up the crowded footpath to the mountaintop resorts. Sunday afternoon, often weary and footsore, the hikers would emerge from the mountains to find the big red cars waiting, ready for the homeward journey.

With the end of the hiking era and the distraction of World War II, the old Mount Wilson Trail fell into years of disuse. Gradually it became overgrown and badly eroded in spots. In 1953 UNSAFE TO

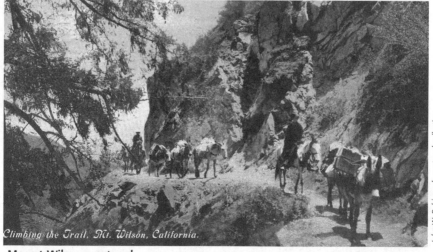

Climbing the Trail. Mt. Wilson, California.

Mount Wilson postcard

John W. Robinson's postcard collection

TRAVEL signs were posted at both ends of the historic pathway. Fortunately, a group of Sierra Madre volunteers, led by Bill Wark, spent many weekends restoring the trail, and it was reopened in 1960. The late Ambrose Zaro maintained the trail for 30 years before his death in 1990.

Description

Drive to the junction of Mira Monte Avenue and Mount Wilson Trail Drive in Sierra Madre. Leave your car in the immediate area of the junction, not up on Mount Wilson Trail Drive.

Walk about 150 yards up Mount Wilson Trail Drive to the beginning of the trail, marked by a large wooden sign. Then follow the trail to Orchard Camp, 3.5 miles (*see* Hike 39). Be sure to fill your water bottle at Orchard

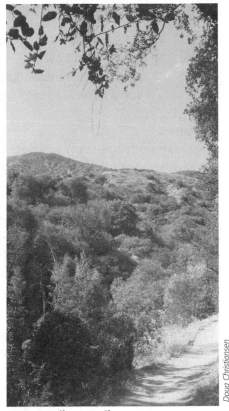

Mount Wilson Trail

Camp; this is the last dependable water. (As always, purify it before drinking.) Follow the trail as it climbs steeply through chaparral, oaks, and firs up the west slope of Little Santa Anita Canyon. The trail crosses the canyon near its head and switches back eastward to the firebreak atop the ridge separating Little Santa Anita from Winter Creek. Here, you intersect the Winter Creek Trail (*see* Hike 44). Turn left (west) and continue up the trail as it zigzags steeply up to the Mount Wilson Toll Road, 2 miles from Orchard Camp. Turn right and follow the old toll road through an open forest to its junction with the Mount Wilson Road just outside the entrance to Skyline Park, 1 mile.

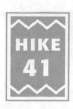

CHANTRY FLAT TO STURTEVANT FALLS

HIKE LENGTH: 3.75 miles round-trip; 500' elevation gain
DIFFICULTY: Easy
SEASON: November–June
TOPO MAP: *Mount Wilson*

Features

Although there are many cascades and small water drops in Big Santa
Anita, Sturtevant Falls is the only real waterfall in the canyon. Its silver spray plunges 50 feet into a shallow, rock-ribbed pool, shaded by
alders and oaks. En route you pass through a beautiful grove of oaks
and ferns at the site of old Fern Lodge. In spring, there are fine displays
of wildflowers, particularly prickly phlox and sticky monkey flower.

This is a short, leisurely stroll from Chantry Flat, a good beginner's hike. You can combine the trip with a picnic under the oaks at
Chantry Flat, where there are stoves, tables, and water.

Description

From the Foothill Freeway in Arcadia, take the Santa Anita Avenue
off-ramp and drive north to Chantry Flat, 5 miles. The Chantry
Flat Road is sometimes closed for repair. Check with the US Forest
Service before attempting this hike. Also note that the gate at the
top of the residential portion of Chantry Flat Road is closed 8 p.m.–
6 a.m.; plan accordingly. Be sure to display your Adventure Pass on
your parked vehicle.

Take the Gabrielino Trail, which descends from the entrance to
Chantry Flat into Big Santa Anita Canyon. Cross the Winter Creek
Bridge and walk up the broad canyon trail, passing numerous private
cabins, to a three-way trail junction. Continue straight ahead. You
ford Big Santa Anita Creek in 200 yards, and then reford where the
canyon makes a sharp bend left. Scramble over boulders the last 100
yards to the large pool at the foot of the falls.

Please do not attempt to climb the falls; people have been injured
trying to do so.

Return the way you came.

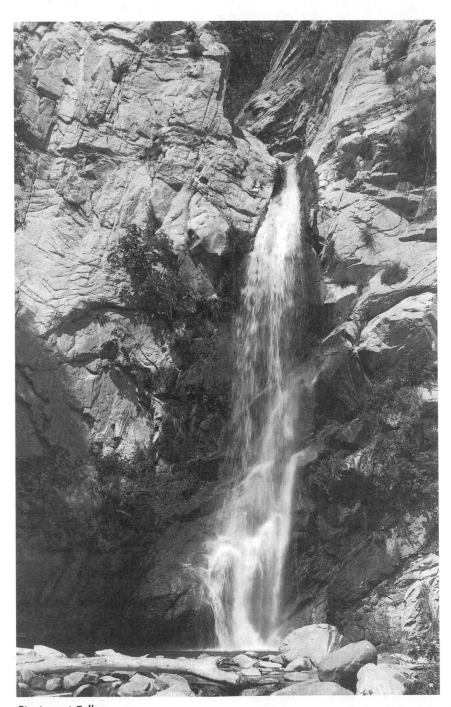

Sturtevant Falls

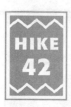

CHANTRY FLAT TO SPRUCE GROVE TRAIL CAMP

HIKE LENGTH: 8 miles round-trip; 1,400' elevation gain
DIFFICULTY: Moderate
SEASON: November–June
TOPO MAP: *Mount Wilson*

Features

Big Santa Anita Canyon is one of the most beautiful wooded glens in
the San Gabriels, a favorite sylvan retreat for nature lovers, hikers,
and campers. Under spreading evergreens, the musical waters of Big
Santa Anita Creek reveal a delightful diversity of moods—now dancing merrily over a pebble-strewn floor, then pausing in a limpid pool,
only to plunge headlong over a waterfall and cascade to begin a new
cycle. Along the banks sprout regal Woodwardia ferns, dotted here
and there in springtime with clusters of lupines, larkspurs, and other
flowering herbs, all contributing to nature's soft picture of elegance.

Detracting somewhat from the primeval scene are the dozens of
check dams, built of precast concrete and interlocked like giant
Lincoln logs, which have converted the once-rustic canyon bottom
into a progression of artificial stairsteps, with glassy sheets of water
pouring over 10- to 20-foot drops. These check dams were constructed by the Los Angeles County Flood Control District and the
US Forest Service in the early 1960s as safeguards against erosion,
much to the disgust of conservationists. Fortunately, 40 years of
nature's regrowth have softened the appearance of artificiality, and
the canyon has regained much of its former beauty.

Big Santa Anita has a rich history. In the 1850s there was a gold
strike in the lower canyon, just about where Santa Anita Dam and
Reservoir are now. The excitement lasted a few years, and then the
miners drifted away. In 1886–1887, the Burlingame brothers constructed a rough road along the west slopes of the canyon to Winter
Creek, intent on hauling out timber to fire their charcoal kilns. But
the San Gabriels were declared a timber reserve before the brothers
could cut any trees. In the 1890s Wilbur M. Sturtevant, one of the
real pioneers in the range, hewed out his famous trail to the head of
the canyon, where he set up Sturtevant's Camp, long one of the most
popular trail resorts in the mountains. Others followed "Sturde." To
cater to the swarms of hikers who visited the canyon every weekend,

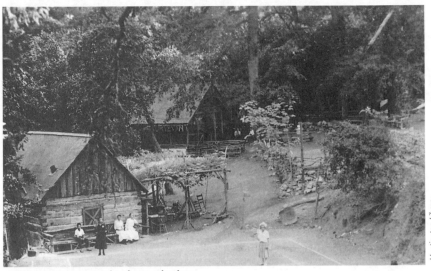

Sturtevant's Camp in the early days

a host of trail hostelries were established—Joe Clark's Halfway House; First Water Camp, where the trail over the ridge from Sierra Madre first touched the stream; Roberts' Camp, at the junction of Big Santa Anita and Winter Creek; Fern Lodge and the Sierra Club's Muir Lodge below Sturtevant Falls; and Hoegees Trail Camp halfway up Winter Creek. All these old camps except Sturtevant's, which is now a church retreat, are gone today.

This very pleasant trip takes you through the lushly forested heart of Big Santa Anita, passing the sites of many of the historic hostelries, to Spruce Grove Trail Camp in the upper canyon.

Description

From the Foothill Freeway in Arcadia, take the Santa Anita Avenue off-ramp and drive north to Chantry Flat, 5 miles. The Chantry Flat Road is sometimes closed for repair. Check with the US Forest Service before attempting this hike. Also note that the gate at the top of the residential portion of Chantry Flat Road is closed 8 p.m.–6 a.m.; plan accordingly. Be sure to display your Adventure Pass on your parked vehicle.

To the right of the road as you enter Chantry Flat, you will notice a locked gate and a paved fire road descending into the canyon. A large sign proclaims this road THE GABRIELINO RECREATION TRAIL (*see* Hike 47) and gives trail mileages. Follow this fire road to the canyon bottom, 0.5 mile, cross the Winter Creek Bridge, and walk up Big Santa Anita Canyon on the broad trail, passing numerous check dams and private cabins. About 0.5 mile farther you enter a shady recess and pass a cluster of cabins, once the site of Fern Lodge. Just beyond, the trail forks three ways: straight ahead to Sturtevant Falls (*see* Hike 41), left and then sharp right up the slope to climb above the falls into the middle canyon, and sharp left up the hillside to the upper canyon. Either of the last two trails may be taken; they rejoin in a mile. The leftmost one is easier walking, while the middle path directly above the falls and through the scenic middle section of the canyon is more beautiful. In 1.5 miles you drop back beside the alder- and bay-shaded stream and reach Cascade Picnic Area, on a forested bench to the right of the creek. Continue up the trail as it climbs the east slope, and then drops to ford the creek and ascends to Spruce Grove Trail Camp, 0.75 mile farther. There are stoves and tables here, the only place in the canyon where you can legally camp. (If possible, do this trip on a weekday; weekends usually find Spruce Grove crowded with Boy Scout campers.)

Return the way you came.

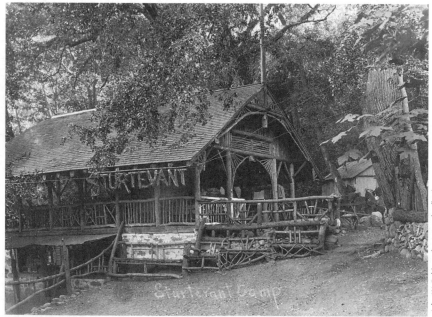

Sturtevant Camp

John W. Robinson's postcard collection

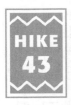

CHANTRY FLAT VIA STURTEVANT TRAIL TO HOEGEES TRAIL CAMP, MOUNT ZION, BIG SANTA ANITA CANYON

HIKE LENGTH: 10 miles round-trip; 1,800' elevation gain
DIFFICULTY: Moderate
SEASON: November–June
TOPO MAP: *Mount Wilson*

Features

This very attractive circle hike follows the old Sturtevant Trail, known today as the Upper Winter Creek Trail, from Chantry Flat to Hoegees Trail Camp, and then climbs over Mount Zion Saddle and drops into upper Big Santa Anita Canyon. You then follow the canyon trail down past Sturtevant Camp, Spruce Grove Trail Camp, and Cascade Picnic Area to lower Winter Creek, and then climb back up to Chantry Flat. This is a delightful circle trip—one of the best in the San Gabriels—passing across chaparral-coated slopes with expansive canyon views, through lush conifer forest and streamside woodland, and alongside bubbling creeks, fully sampling the grandeur of the Big Santa Anita watershed.

Wilbur Sturtevant, known as "Sturdy" to his friends, built his trail from Sierra Madre over the ridge into Big Santa Anita Canyon, and then along the west slope to his resort camp in 1896. For decades, the famous Sturtevant Trail felt the trod of many boots and the joyous voices of legions of hikers bound for the delights of Big Santa Anita and its many hostelries of the Great Hiking Era. One who hiked the Sturtevant Trail and fell in love with alder-and-fern-lined Winter Creek was Arie Hoegee, who built his resort camp there in 1908. For three decades it was a favorite destination for hikers. The rustic buildings are long gone, but the US Forest Service has made the little streamside glen into Hoegees Trail Camp, with stoves and tables. Hoegees Trail Camp has an unusual distinction: in the 24-hour period of January 22–23, 1942, a total of 26.12 inches of rain fell here, establishing a Southern California record that still stands.

Description

From Foothill Freeway in Arcadia, take the Santa Anita Avenue off-ramp and drive north to Chantry Flat, 5 miles. The Chantry Flat Road is sometimes closed for repair, so check with the US Forest Service before attempting this hike. Note that the gate at the top of the residential portion of Chantry Flat Road is closed 8 p.m.–6 a.m.; plan accordingly. Be sure to display your Adventure Pass on your parked vehicle.

From the upper parking area at Chantry Flat, take the fire road that begins to the left (south) of the ranger station, adjacent to the sloping picnic area. After 0.25 mile, at the road's second switchback, turn right onto the Upper Winter Creek Trail, indicated by a wooden sign. Follow the trail as it climbs, contours, and then drops along the west wall of Big Santa Anita Canyon, mostly through chaparral, passing a Mount Wilson Trail junction to Winter Creek in 2 miles. Your trail fords Winter Creek, briefly climbs, and then drops to another trail junction. For Hoegees Trail Camp, go right; the trail refords Winter Creek and reaches the tree-shaded camp after a few minutes' walk. (An option that cuts your hiking distance in half is to descend the Winter Creek Trail to the Big Santa Anita Canyon Trail, and then turn right and climb back up to Chantry Flat.)

To continue on the full circle trip, retrace your steps from Hoegees Trail Camp back up to the Mount Zion Trail junction, marked by a small sign. Go right and follow the newly restored Mount Zion Trail (which is really the upper section of the old Sturtevant Trail) as it climbs, first through forest and then chaparral, to Zion Saddle, 1.25 miles. A side trail right leads 0.25 mile to Mount Zion's summit and spectacular views over the Big Santa Anita watershed. Your main trail then gently descends through lush forest, mostly big-cone Douglas-firs, to a junction with the Big Santa Anita Canyon Trail, 0.75 mile. Turn right and descend the canyon trail, fording the creek twice, to Spruce Grove Trail Camp, 0.5 mile. Your trail descends to Cascade Picnic Area, contours the mountainside, drops to Winter Creek, and climbs back up to Chantry Flat (*see* Hike 42 for a full description).

Note: This circle trip was made possible by the restoration of the Mount Zion section of the Sturtevant Trail by Howard Casey, Chris Kasten, and Bohdan Porendowski of Camp Sturtevant in 1976–1979, and The Big Santa Anita Gang and Sierra Club volunteers in 1984–1985.

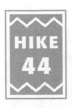

CHANTRY FLAT TO MOUNT WILSON VIA WINTER CREEK

HIKE LENGTH: 7 miles one way; 3,600' elevation gain
DIFFICULTY: Strenuous
SEASON: November–June
TOPO MAP: *Mount Wilson*

Features

Mount Wilson can be climbed by trails from more directions than any other peak in Southern California. The mountain is laced with footpaths.

This trail goes from Chantry Flat over the old Sturtevant Trail to Winter Creek, and then climbs steeply up through a dense forest of big-cone Douglas-firs and oaks to the Winter Creek–Little Santa Anita divide, where it joins the Old Mount Wilson Trail and continues on to the toll road and the summit. A number of interesting variations can be planned (see below). Be in top physical shape; the trip is steeply uphill most of the way.

Description

From the Foothill Freeway in Arcadia, take the Santa Anita Avenue off-ramp and drive north to Chantry Flat, 5 miles. The Chantry Flat Road is sometimes closed for repair. Check with the US Forest Service before attempting this hike. Also note that the gate on Chantry Flat Road is closed 8 p.m.–6 a.m.; get an early start. Be sure to display your Adventure Pass on your parked vehicle.

Walk from the parking area up to the Chantry Flat Ranger Station, and start up the fire road that begins 50 feet left (south) of it, adjacent to the sloping picnic area. After a short 0.25-mile trip, at the road's second switchback, turn right (northwest) onto the Sturtevant Trail (marked UPPER WINTER CREEK TRAIL on the topo map) and follow it around the ridges 1.5 miles to a trail junction where a sign indicates Mount Wilson. If you reach Winter Creek above Hoegees Trail Camp, you've gone 100 yards too far. Turn left (northwest) at the junction and follow the trail as it climbs steeply for 2 miles through firs and oaks to the ridgetop and a second trail junction. Here, you intersect the Old Mount Wilson Trail coming up from Little Santa Anita Canyon (*see* Hike 40). Continue up the ridgetop trail as it zigzags steeply up, back and forth across the firebreak, to the Mount

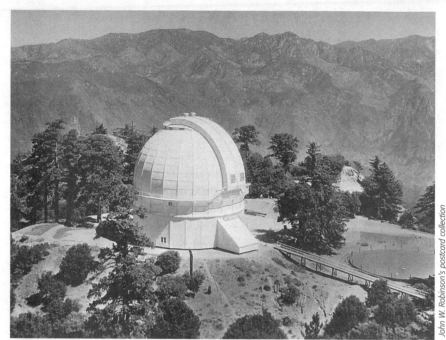

John W. Robinson's postcard collection

Mount Wilson Observatory

Wilson Toll Road, 0.5 mile farther. Turn right and follow the old toll road 1 mile through open stands of evergreens to its junction with the Mount Wilson Road just outside the entrance to Skyline Park.

You have several options on this trip. You can descend the way you came up. You can have someone waiting for you at the road loop outside Mount Wilson Skyline Park to drive you down. You can descend the old toll road to Altadena (*see* Hike 27) or the Old Mount Wilson Trail via Little Santa Anita Canyon to Sierra Madre (*see* Hike 40)—both of these options require a car shuttle. Or you can enter Skyline Park (open April 1–November 30; with refreshments available Friday–Sunday, 10 a.m.–5 p.m.), walk past the observatory grounds to the east end of the mountain, and descend via the Sturtevant Trail (*see* Hike 45).

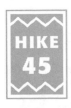

CHANTRY FLAT TO STURTEVANT CAMP AND MOUNT WILSON

HIKE LENGTH: 8 miles one way; 3,900' elevation gain
DIFFICULTY: Strenuous
SEASON: November–June
TOPO MAP: *Mount Wilson*

Features

The canyon of Big Santa Anita cuts a deep semicircular groove into the south flank of the front range, its head lying close under the precipitous east slope of Mount Wilson. An old trail travels most of the length of the canyon, and then switchbacks steeply up forest- and chaparral-covered slopes to the mountaintop. For many years the pathway was overgrown and eroded, but recently it has been reworked and put in good condition—steep but easily passable.

This trip follows this old route, traveling up-canyon from Chantry Flat to Sturtevant Camp, and then climbing right up the mountainside to Echo Rock and the observatory grounds. It is long and tiring; be in top shape. For the descent, you have a number of options; see the Description below.

Description

From the Foothill Freeway in Arcadia, take the Santa Anita Avenue off-ramp and drive the 5 miles north to Chantry Flat. The Chantry Flat Road is sometimes closed for repair. Check with the US Forest Service before attempting this hike. Be aware that the gate on Chantry Flat Road is closed 8 p.m.–6 a.m.; plan accordingly. Be sure to display your Adventure Pass on your parked vehicle.

Take the fire road that descends from near the entrance of Chantry Flat into Big Santa Anita, and then follow the canyon trail to Spruce Grove Trail Camp, 4 miles (*see* Hike 42). Your trail climbs above the camp, fords the stream, and reaches a trail junction, the right fork going up to Newcomb Pass and on into the West Fork country (*see* Hike 46). Go left above the creek; almost immediately, you reach the woodsy haunt of Sturtevant Camp, operated as a Methodist Church retreat. Just before entering the camp, your trail turns sharply left and crosses the creek just above a debris barrier. You now leave the canyon and switchback steeply up through dense forest cover, which thins as you get higher, to Echo Rock at the east end of the Mount

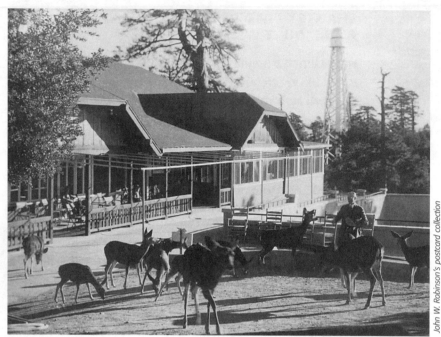

Mount Wilson Hotel (circa 1930)

Wilson summit plateau, 8 miles from Chantry Flat. Walk through the observatory grounds to Skyline Park.

From the summit, you have several options. You can descend the way you came. You can cross the Mount Wilson Observatory grounds and Skyline Park to the one-way, exit-only gate at Skyline Park and have someone waiting for you at the road loop. You can descend the old toll road to Altadena (*see* Hike 27) or the Old Mount Wilson Trail via Little Santa Anita Canyon to Sierra Madre (*see* Hike 40)—both of these options require a car shuttle. Or you can descend the Winter Creek Trail back to Chantry Flat (*see* Hike 44). This last alternative is suggested; it makes for an interesting and strenuous circle trip with no car shuttle.

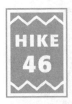

CHANTRY FLAT TO NEWCOMB PASS, WEST FORK OF THE SAN GABRIEL RIVER, DEVORE TRAIL CAMP, WEST FORK CAMPGROUND

HIKE LENGTH: 9 miles one way; 2,300' elevation gain
DIFFICULTY: Strenuous
SEASON: November–June
TOPO MAP: *Mount Wilson*

Features

Big Santa Anita was once the gateway into the San Gabriel backcountry, before the Angeles Crest Highway tamed the range and forever changed it. Anglers, hunters, and adventurers by the score tramped up the Sturtevant Trail, over the divide at Newcomb Pass, and into the wild interior of the range.

In 1896 Wilbur Sturtevant completed his trail into his resort camp near the head of the canyon. Louie Newcomb, another mountain pioneer who had settled in Chilao around 1888, decided that "Sturde's" footpath would make an excellent first leg for trips into his beloved backcountry. So with the help of 10 laborers, Newcomb thrashed out a rough pathway over the divide that now bears his name—Newcomb Pass—and down into the West Fork, and then up Shortcut Canyon and on to his Chilao country. While Newcomb was working on his path, Sturtevant and several others incorporated the Sierra Madre and Antelope Valley Toll Trail and charged 25¢ per person to hike across the range to the desert, with the first fares going to Newcomb for his part in building the trail. However, Newcomb, who had to do the collecting himself, complained that no system of collecting would work without someone on the trail at all times, and "that don't pay wages, so I had to quit it." So passed a brief and colorful episode in the story of San Gabriel trails. Although the toll was abandoned, the trail remained, and for three decades—until the completion of the Angeles Crest in the mid-1930s—it was a major thoroughfare for backcountry ramblers.

Today a network of paved highways and unpaved byways provides easy access to the mountain regions behind Mount Wilson. The once-vital trail over Newcomb Pass is virtually unused. But this pathway hewed by Newcomb a century ago remains; in fact it has recently been worked and is in good condition.

This trip no longer leads to wild mountain recesses as it once did, but it traverses some scenic chaparral and pine country in its long course from Chantry Flat over the historic divide and down to old West Fork Campground. From there, you can explore a number of interesting options, described below.

Description

From the Foothill Freeway in Arcadia, take the Santa Anita Avenue off-ramp and drive north to Chantry Flat, 5 miles. The Chantry Flat Road is sometimes closed for repair, so check with the US Forest Service before attempting this hike. Also, be aware that the gate on Chantry Flat Road is closed 8 p.m.–6 a.m.; plan accordingly.

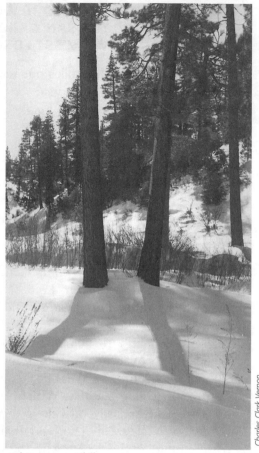

Charles Clark Vernon

Winter near Chilao

Be sure to display your Adventure Pass on your parked vehicle.

Take the fire road that descends from near the entrance of Chantry Flat into Big Santa Anita, and then follow the canyon trail to Spruce Grove Campground, 4 miles. Less than 0.5 mile beyond the campground, just before you reach Sturtevant Camp, is a trail junction. Go right (northeast) up the slope and around the chaparral-rich ridges to Newcomb Pass, a long 2 miles (a sign at the pass says 3). Here, you meet a fire road coming in from the east; do not take it. Continue north on the trail, switchbacking down through a forest of firs and oaks and crossing the Rincon–Red Box fire road after a short 0.25 mile, for 2 miles to Devore Trail Camp on the West Fork. Although the 2009 Station Fire incinerated the slopes just north of here, the canyon bottom fared better and retains its woodsy charm. From Devore the trail becomes overgrown and difficult to follow in places, requiring several stream crossings. In a mile you reach shady West Fork Campground and the dirt road coming down from Red Box.

You now have a number of options. You can return the way you came. You can walk a mile up the road toward Red Box, and then take the Kenyon Devore Trail up Mount Wilson (*see* Hike 51) and descend back to Chantry Flat via either the trail down the head of Big Santa Anita (*see* Hike 45) or the toll road–Winter Creek Trail (*see* Hike 44). Or you can continue on the route of Louie Newcomb and the backcountry pioneers, taking the trail up Shortcut Canyon to the Angeles Crest (*see* Hike 53), and then down into the upper Big Tujunga, up to Charlton Flat and on to Chilao. This totals 18 miles, necessitating an overnight stay at either Devore Trail Camp or West Fork Campground.

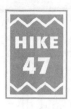

GABRIELINO NATIONAL RECREATION TRAIL

HIKE LENGTH: 28 miles one way; 4,800' elevation gain
DIFFICULTY: Strenuous (2 days); moderate (3–4 days)
SEASON: November–June
TOPO MAPS: *Mount Wilson, Chilao Flat, Condor Peak, Pasadena*

Features

Note: The portion of the trail covered in day three—the stretch from Switzer's down the Arroyo Seco to Oakwilde—is, as of this writing (spring 2013), closed to entry due to the 2009 Station Fire. Check with the US Forest Service for updates before attempting this last portion of the hike.

The Gabrielino National Recreation Trail was established by the US Forest Service in 1970 as an outgrowth of the National Trails System Act passed by Congress. "This trail has been created for you—the city dweller—so that you might exchange, for a short time, the hectic scene of your urban life for the rugged beauty and freedom of adventure into the solitary wonderland of nature"—so said a US Forest Service bulletin announcing the new trail. Actually the trail is not new; it is a joining together and reworking of several old footpaths to form a semicircle over and around the central part of the front range. The route covered in this trip starts at Chantry Flat and goes to Big Santa Anita Canyon, Newcomb Pass, West Fork of San Gabriel River, Red Box, and Arroyo Seco, and it finishes at Altadena. En route you sample the varied terrain and vegetation found in the front range: oak-shaded canyons, fir- and pine-dotted mountainsides, and chaparral-coated lower slopes. And, particularly on the portion up to Red Box, you will transit areas that were severely burned in the Station Fire. You can camp overnight at any of six US Forest Service campgrounds on the circular route.

The name commemorates the Gabrielino Indians, who roamed these mountains long before the arrival of the white settlers in Southern California. These peaceful people migrated into the mountain canyons of the San Gabriels every summer to gather acorns and hunt wild game.

This trip is best done as a three- or four-day backpack trip. If you're in a monumental hurry, you can do it in two long days.

Description

Drive to Chantry Flat, 5 miles up Santa Anita Avenue from Arcadia. This road sometimes closes unexpectedly; check with the US Forest Service to make sure it's open. Note that the gate on Chantry Flat Road is closed 8 p.m.–6 a.m. Arrange to be picked up at the foot of the Arroyo Seco Trail, at the intersection of Ventura Street and Windsor Avenue in Altadena. The description below is of a three-day outing. You can vary the trip to suit your own hiking pace and inclination.

Day 1: Hike from Chantry Flat up the Big Santa Anita Canyon Trail, passing the first trail camp at Spruce Grove, and continue over Newcomb Pass and down to Devore Trail Camp on the West Fork of the San Gabriel River, 9 miles (*see* Hike 46). Spend your first night here, or 1 mile farther at the West Fork Public Campground. If you get a late start from Chantry Flat, you can stay the night at Spruce Grove Trail Camp, 4 miles up Big Santa Anita Canyon, adding an extra half day to the trip.

Day 2: Hike up the West Fork to Red Box, 6 miles. The easy-graded pathway follows the main creek from Devore Trail Camp to West Fork Campground—this 1-mile stretch is overgrown and difficult to follow in places, and then climbs along the south slope, several hundred feet above the stream, before finally zigzagging up to Red Box Saddle. Here, you will see the unmistakable effects of the 2009 Station Fire, which drastically altered the character of this once-lush portion of the trail. Then you drop into the head of the Arroyo Seco. The trail starts at the northwest edge of the Red Box parking area and descends to Commodore Switzer Trail Camp, 4.5 miles. This comes to 10.5 miles for the day. Spend your second night here.

Day 3: Descend the Arroyo Seco Trail to Oakwilde (*see* Hike 16) and on down the canyon to Altadena (*see* Hike 15), 8.5 miles.

If you desire to do the trip in two days, the best overnight camp is Valley Forge Campground, midway up the West Fork. This will give you 12 miles of hiking the first day, and a long 16 miles on the second. Remember, you must camp in one of the authorized campgrounds.

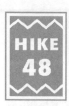

MONROVIA CANYON PARK TO SAWPIT CANYON, DEER PARK

HIKE 48

HIKE LENGTH: 6.5 miles round-trip; 1,100' elevation gain
DIFFICULTY: Moderate
SEASON: All year
TOPO MAPS: *Mount Wilson, Azusa*

Features

Beautiful Sawpit Canyon drains the southern slopes of Monrovia Peak. A lush canopy of alders and bays lines the creek, and the slopes are blanketed with a thick cover of chaparral and, in the shadier recesses, oaks and big-cone Douglas-firs. The city lies just over the ridge to the south, but here, you're in another world.

This very pleasant trip begins at the lower end of Monrovia Canyon Park, follows the fire road up around Sawpit Canyon Reservoir, and then ascends the Overturff Trail to a little oak-shaded flat tucked into the south ramparts of Monrovia Peak known as Deer Park. The shady recess was discovered by Monrovia building contractor Ben Overturff around 1905. He built a stone cabin there, and for many years, from 1911 to the 1938 flood, Deer Park Lodge was a popular trail resort. Only the foundations remain today, under a canopy of majestic canyon oaks with a delightful all-year stream nearby.

You must pay a $5 admission fee to enter Monrovia Canyon Park. Hours are Monday–Friday, 8 a.m.–5 p.m., and Saturday–Sunday, 7 a.m.–5 p.m. The park is closed Tuesday, when the Monrovia Police Department uses its Sawpit Canyon Shooting Range.

Description

Leave the Foothill Freeway (I-210) at Myrtle Avenue in Monrovia. Drive north on Myrtle, through town, 2 miles to Scenic Drive. Turn right and follow the latter, with short jogs right, and then left, curving north as Scenic Drive becomes Canyon Boulevard, to the Monrovia Canyon Park entrance station. Pay your fee and park in the lower parking area opposite the signed trailhead.

Walk steeply up the Sawpit Canyon fire road, passing Sawpit Dam, built by the Los Angeles County Flood Control District in 1929, and, farther up, Trask Boy Scout Camp, both to your left. The road becomes unpaved just past the dam. After a mile, the road curves

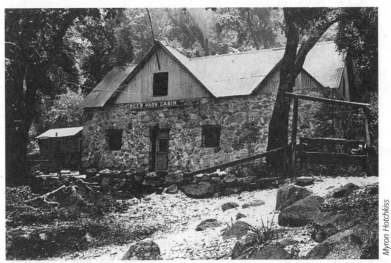

Deer Park Cabin (circa 1925)

left and you reach the lower end of the Overturff Trail on your left, marked by a sign and two low stone pillars.

Follow the trail as it descends to Sawpit Creek, crosses it, and climbs to the Razorback, a sharp divide separating Sycamore and Sawpit Canyons. You follow the crest of the Razorback a short distance, and then climb the chaparral-covered slope to The Gap, a break in the ridge. Beyond, your pathway descends, contours, and gently climbs beneath a shady canopy of oaks and bay laurels. You reach Twin Springs Creek, where flowing water from one of the springs has formed a natural bridge. Just across the creek you pass a junction with a lateral trail that drops down to Sawpit Canyon fire road. You take the main trail straight ahead, climb over a low ridge, cross Deer Park Creek, and reach a second junction. Go left and climb 100 yards to Deer Park. Only the foundations remain of the once-popular lodge, shaded by tall oaks. It's a nice picnic spot. Return the way you came, or drop down either of the two short lateral trails to Sawpit Canyon fire road and follow the latter back to your car.

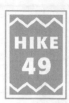

DUARTE TO MOUNT BLISS
VIA VAN TASSEL FIRE ROAD

HIKE LENGTH: 8.5 miles round-trip; 2,900' elevation gain
SEASON: November–May
DIFFICULTY: Moderate
TOPO MAPS: *Mount Wilson, Azusa*

Features

What later became known as the Great Fire of 1924 began in September of that year in San Gabriel Canyon and burned for more than two weeks, devastating the front range of the San Gabriels and for a time threatening the city of Monrovia. Rush Charlton, superintendent of the Angeles National Forest at the time, commented, "The greatest difficulty in fighting the fire was the lack of roads over which to transport supplies to the men." In response, the US Forest Service began a crash course to design and build a series of access roads and firebreaks intended to help prevent a recurrence of the 1924 holocaust. Today the results of that effort are seen in the score of dirt roadways—fire roads—that crisscross the range, especially at the lower elevations.

One such road is the Van Tassel fire road, also called the Silver Fish Truck Trail on some maps. This trip follows its lower portion and samples the chaparral-blanketed slopes high above Duarte and Monrovia as it climbs steeply up to 3,720-foot Mount Bliss and, on a clear day, a 360-degree panoramic view over the surrounding mountains and the valley below. Like almost all of the front range fire roads, it is virtually shadeless and should not be done in warm weather.

Description

From the Foothill Freeway (I-210), take the Irwindale Avenue off-ramp. Drive north to Foothill Boulevard and turn left (west). Follow Foothill, which becomes Huntington Drive, to Encanto Parkway, 1 mile. Turn right (north) on Encanto Parkway and drive 1.3 miles to the entrance to Encanto Equestrian Center; turn left and follow the dirt road 0.5 mile to its end. Park along the left side of the road, across from the horse stables. An Adventure Pass is not needed to park here.

From the parking area, walk north and follow the fire road as it curves to the left and climbs steeply above the equestrian center and begins winding its way uphill. In several places the trail traverses saddles affording excellent views of the San Gabriel Valley immediately to the south. After just under 4 miles of steady climbing, Mount Bliss comes into view ahead; you pass under some power lines and reach a junction with a service road that branches off to the right. Take this service road, and after 100 feet, look for a narrow use trail leading to the left through the shrubbery; follow it a short distance up to a ridge and continue on to the summit.

After enjoying the view, return the way you came. Or, for an excellent one-way trip, continue north on the fire road 1.5 miles farther to White Saddle; turn left and descend into Sawpit Canyon, and then join and follow the Overturff Trail to Monrovia Canyon Park (*see* Hike 48). This option, totaling 10.5 miles, requires an 8-mile car shuttle between Azusa and Monrovia.

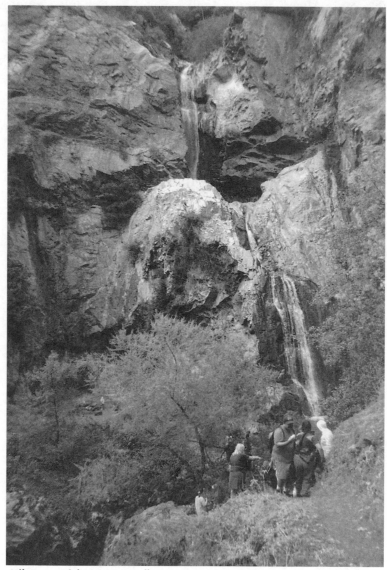

Hikers at Fish Canyon Falls

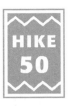

AZUSA TO FISH CANYON, FISH CANYON FALLS

HIKE LENGTH: 4 miles round-trip; 500' elevation gain
DIFFICULTY: Easy
SEASON: Winter–summer subject to access
TOPO MAP: *Azusa*

Features

Fish Canyon Falls are some of the top natural attractions of the San Gabriel Mountains. In spring, when the water runs high, the falls are a spectacular delight, plunging some 80 feet in stairway fashion. The topmost fall is the longest, shooting out from the narrow gorge above, and then swishing down into a sparkling pool 40 feet below. Then there is a short cascade, followed by a 30-foot plunge into a lower pool, with one final 8-foot drop below that. A fine silver spray dampens the canyon walls when the water runs high, causing the walls to be embossed with lush green mosses and grasses. In the amphitheater below, aroar with the boom of the falls, there is a small flat, shaded by oaks and overhanging rock—a favorite spot of picnickers.

For decades, the canyon entrance was blocked by the quarrying operation of the Vulcan Materials Company. To circumnavigate this obstacle, a steep trail, poorly built in places, was constructed in 1998. The footpath climbs 1,600 feet up the west slope of the canyon, and then drops 1,200 feet back into the canyon just upstream from the quarry, all to travel a linear mile! This tortuous, unmaintained route is *not* recommended.

To their credit, Vulcan Materials has designated several Saturdays each year—beginning in winter or spring and running through August—as open-access days during which transit through its property to the trail is permitted. A free shuttle is provided to deliver hikers to the trailhead and then back again. This is the only sensible way to hike Fish Canyon. For a list of applicable dates, visit the website at **azusarock.com**.

Description

From the Foothill Freeway (I-210), take the Irwindale Avenue off-ramp. Drive north to Foothill Boulevard and turn left (west). Follow Foothill, which becomes Huntington Drive, to Encanto Parkway, 1 mile. Turn right (north) on Encanto Parkway and drive 1.75 miles to Vulcan Materials' main gate; free parking is available inside the gate on the designated open-access days. Shuttles to the trailhead begin running at 7 a.m.; the last return shuttle leaves at 3 p.m.

Once you leave the quarry behind, this becomes a delightful hike. Your trail contours along the west slope about 50 feet above the creek, shaded by a canopy of live oaks, big-leaf maples, and alders. You pass the foundations of several cabin remains, and then switchback higher up the canyon slope before dropping to the creek, 1.5 miles in. You cross a small tributary stream, and then the main creek, and ascend the east slope to a sharp bend in the canyon where the falls abruptly come into view. Carefully descend the rocky slope to a shaded amphitheater alongside a shallow pool, just beneath the falls. Do not attempt to climb the falls, even though the rocks to the left look inviting. People have been severely injured trying.

Return the way you came. Years ago, a trail climbed up the east slope around the falls and continued up Fish Canyon to Stone Cabin Flat, but it has long been abandoned and is now impassable.

If you are a die-hard bent on hiking the punishing trail that climbs around the Vulcan Materials site, leave your car in the dirt parking lot 0.25 mile prior to the Vulcan gate. This trail is narrow, steep, and overgrown in places and should only be attempted by hikers in excellent physical condition. Do it on a cool, cloudy, winter day, and bring ample water.

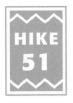

MOUNT WILSON VIA KENYON DEVORE TRAIL TO WEST FORK CAMPGROUND

HIKE LENGTH: 9 miles round-trip;
2,800' elevation gain and loss
DIFFICULTY: Moderate
SEASON: All year
TOPO MAP: *Mount Wilson*

Features

Kenyon DeVore (1911–1995) spent his whole life in and around the San Gabriel Mountains. He grew up at his parents' trail resorts on the West Fork of the San Gabriel River, first at Camp West Fork and then at Valley Forge Lodge. As a child, he busied himself with camp chores. As a teenager, he worked at the Mount Wilson Hotel and led a pack train that supplied resorts, forest stations, and campers throughout the mountains. DeVore spent most of his adult life working for the Los Angeles County Flood Control District, most of the time in San Gabriel Canyon. After his retirement in 1971, he signed on as an Angeles National Forest volunteer, and later as a part-time paid employee. For 15 years he was a familiar sight at the Chantry Flat visitor information station, giving advice and imparting knowledge to hikers, backpackers, and picnickers. It was only fitting that the old Rattlesnake Trail, which DeVore traveled many times with his pack train, be renamed in his honor.

The Kenyon DeVore Trail descends Strayns Creek from Mount Wilson to the West Fork of the San Gabriel. Despite its tortuous and coiling route down the very steep canyon, it is one of the best trail trips in the San Gabriels. Situated entirely on a north-facing slope (the other Mount Wilson trails approach from the south or the east), the path runs through lush forest all the way—Jeffrey and sugar pines, incense cedars, big-cone Douglas-firs, and many stands of oaks. Except for a portion near and along a section of the West Fork, damage from the 2009 Station Fire is minimal. Even on a warm day, this well-shaded trip is enjoyable. You cross Strayns Creek several times; in spring and early summer, the trickling water is ice cold and refreshing (but filter it).

Strayns Canyon and Creek were named for A. G. Strain, who operated a resort camp near the upper head of the canyon 1889–1917. The U.S. Geological Survey misspelled his name on the topo sheet, and the mistake has never been corrected.

Description

Drive up the Angeles Crest Highway to Red Box, 14 miles from La Cañada. Turn right and follow Mount Wilson Road to near the summit, 4 miles. The Kenyon DeVore Trail begins 0.25 mile west of the summit, where the pavement splits and becomes one-way. Park in a large clearing south of the road or drive around the loop to a smaller clearing on the north side. Be sure to display your Adventure Pass on your parked vehicle.

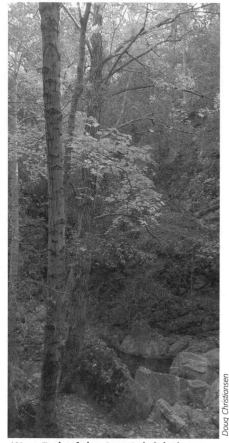

West Fork of the San Gabriel River

The trail drops north through an oak forest along the west slope of Strayns Canyon. You switchback down through open stands of pines, cross the creek, and contour high along the east slope before switchbacking down to the creek and fording it again to the west slope. Then you descend through a shady pine forest, recross Strayns Creek, and drop to a junction with the Gabrielino Trail, 3 miles. Most of the trees in this section were burned away in 2009; you pass through the charred stumps of what used to be forest. Follow the trail east, along the south slope of the canyon, down to West Fork Campground, 1 mile. Here, the fire damage is mostly confined to the slopes north of the stream; the campground remains a sylvan delight. The campground has stoves, tables, and toilets. It is reached by dirt road from Red Box, but as of this writing the road is closed to public autos.

Return the way you came.

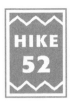

MOUNT WILSON TO WEST FORK CAMPGROUND, DEVORE TRAIL CAMP

HIKE LENGTH: 11 miles round-trip;
2,900' elevation gain and loss
DIFFICULTY: Strenuous (1 day); moderate (2 days)
SEASON: All year
TOPO MAP: *Mount Wilson*

Features

The West Fork of the San Gabriel River—especially the upper part, tucked in behind Mount Wilson—is a delight to anglers, campers, and hikers alike. An all-year stream travels the length of the long canyon, shaded most of the way under oaks, bays, maples, and alders. It offers woodsy haunts and streamside solitude to any who will seek these qualities. The 2009 Station Fire left its mark—particularly in the upper, western portion—but the area remains well worth visiting.

This loop trip, best done as an overnight backpack, drops down from Mount Wilson and samples the best the West Fork has to offer—the shady streamside stretch between West Fork Campground and Devore Trail Camp.

Both of these places are rich in history. Adjacent to West Fork Campground, mountain pioneer Louie Newcomb hand-hewed a log cabin in 1900 that was the first ranger station in California and the second in the United States constructed with government funds ($70). Only the foundation remains today; the old ranger station was disassembled in 1982 and moved to Chilao, where it has been reassembled as a forestry museum behind the Chilao Visitor Center. Devore Trail Camp stands at the site of old Camp West Fork, a small wilderness resort set up by Ernest and Cherie DeVore in 1913. Camp West Fork was a favorite of anglers, most of whom made the trip in via the Sturtevant Trail from Sierra Madre over Newcomb Pass. It was also popular with hikers as a takeoff point for trips into the backcountry. The camp was abandoned after an ownership dispute in 1925, and now nothing remains of the old hostelry. The US Forest Service has made the sylvan site into a trail camp, with stoves, tables, and little flats for sleeping.

Make this a two-day trip, staying a night at either West Fork Campground or Devore Trail Camp, enjoying the gentle murmur of the stream and the soft rustle of leaves in the afternoon breeze.

Note: West Fork Campground is reached by dirt road from Red Box, and the road is closed indefinitely to public vehicular travel.

Description

Drive to the head of the Kenyon DeVore Trail on Mount Wilson Road. Be sure to display your Adventure Pass on your parked vehicle. Walk the 4.5 miles down to West Fork Campground as per Hike 51.

From West Fork Campground cross to the north side of the creek and follow the trail—overgrown and difficult to follow in places—downstream (east) under a forest canopy of oaks, alders, maples, and bays, to Devore Trail Camp, 1 mile. The camp lies on a shady bench on the south side of the creek.

An old anglers' trail continues down the West Fork to Cogswell Reservoir, 5 miles. A few years ago Sierra Club volunteers reworked the first mile of this trail below Devore Trail Camp. The last 4 miles may someday be reworked, but they are overgrown and difficult to follow. Nevertheless, this section of the West Fork contains some of the most beautiful streamside woodlands in the San Gabriels. Sample any part of them you can.

To return from Devore Trail Camp via the recommended loop route, climb steeply south up the Gabrielino Trail, crossing the Red Box–Rincon fire road, to Newcomb Pass on the divide between the West Fork and Big Santa Anita watersheds, 3 miles. Then go right (west) and follow Mount Wilson's Rim Trail, a historic pathway recently restored thanks to the efforts of CORBA, the Concerned Off-Road Bicyclists Association, to the summit. Walk through the observatory grounds out the west gate to your car at the Kenyon DeVore Trail.

Note: The trip should not be made immediately after a heavy rainstorm. The usually serene West Fork can turn into a raging torrent, unsafe to cross.

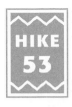

ANGELES CREST HIGHWAY VIA SHORTCUT CANYON TO WEST FORK CAMPGROUND

HIKE LENGTH: 6 miles round-trip;
1,800' elevation gain and loss
DIFFICULTY: Moderate
SEASON: November–May
TOPO MAPS: *Chilao Flat, Mount Wilson*

Features

Years ago, before the Angeles Crest Highway was a reality, Shortcut Canyon felt the trod of many boots and hooves. Its busy trail, built in 1893 by Louie Newcomb, Arthur Carter, and John Hartwell, was the major route into the Charlton Flat–Chilao–Buckhorn backcountry. The canyon and trail were so named because they greatly cut the distance into the mountain interior. The old route was the steep American Indian footpath up Valley Forge Canyon and over Barley Flats, now completely disappeared. Today although the old Shortcut pathway is no longer a major artery of travel, it is part of the Boy Scouts' Silver Moccasin Trail across the range from Red Box to Mount Baden–Powell (*see* page 250). For this reason, the trail is well traveled.

This trip now runs from the top down because the West Fork road from Red Box to West Fork Campground is closed to public autos. Another change is that the historic West Fork Ranger Station, built in 1900 and second-oldest in the nation, has been moved to the Chilao Visitor Center. The evidence of the 2009 Station Fire is all around; most of the surrounding mountainside was burned. Lower down though, along the stream, the West Fork still retains its charm of yesteryear. You will get the feel of the old San Gabriels when bandits, hunters, anglers, and prospectors rambled into the then-wild heart of the range. Most of this hike is now shadeless—due to the fire—so do it on a cool day and bring plenty of water.

Description

Drive up the Angeles Crest Highway to Shortcut Saddle, 19 miles from La Cañada and 0.6 mile past the turnoff for the Upper Big Tujunga Canyon Road, located at highway mileage marker 43.30. Park along either side of the highway. Be sure to display your Adventure Pass on your parked vehicle.

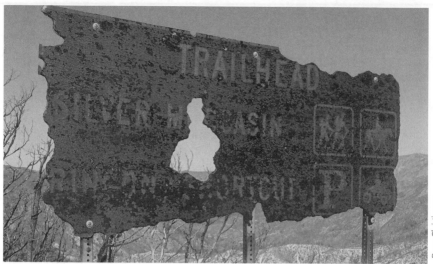

Doug Christiansen

Scorched sign at Shortcut Saddle

From the east side of the saddle, take the unmarked Shortcut Canyon Trail, which leads south. After several short switchbacks you reach a fire road; turn right (west) and follow the fire road about 200 yards, to where you again pick up the trail leading down to your left. Watch carefully for this unmarked junction; it is easy to miss. You drop steeply down fire-ravaged slopes into the East Fork of Shortcut Canyon. Your path now descends the shady canyon floor and passes the junction of Shortcut's West Fork as you cross and recross the trickling creek. After 3 miles you reach the broad West Fork of the San Gabriel. Boulder-hop across the creek (this can be dangerous in times of high water) and reach West Fork Campground, located on a forested bench south of the stream. The campground has stoves, tables, and toilets.

From here, you have several options. One mile down the West Fork is Devore Trail Camp (*see* Hike 52). With a car shuttle you can ascend the Kenyon DeVore Trail to Mount Wilson (*see* Hike 51), or proceed up the Gabrielino Trail to Red Box (*see* Hike 47). Or simply relax a few hours along the canopied creek before heading back up Shortcut Canyon to your car.

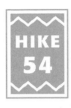

ANGELES FOREST HIGHWAY TO BIG TUJUNGA NARROWS

HIKE LENGTH: 4 miles round-trip;
400' elevation gain and loss
DIFFICULTY: Moderate
SEASON: All year
TOPO MAP: *Condor Peak*

Features

Note: This area is currently closed to entry due to the 2009 Station Fire. Do not attempt this hike until checking with the US Forest Service to verify the current status of the closure.

Big Tujunga Narrows is one of the more spectacular canyons of the San Gabriel range. Precipitous, rock-ribbed, with turbulent white-water hurrying through its shaded bowels, it is exceeded in grandeur only by the East Fork of the San Gabriel River. Although hundreds cross the gorge every day via the Angeles Forest Highway's arched bridge, erected in 1941, only a handful venture down into its cavernous depths. This trip takes you through the heart of the Narrows, first via an exceedingly steep footpath, and then by boulder-hopping alongside the tumultuous stream. Although you're right below a well-traveled highway, the scene is as wild as you can find in the Angeles. One word of warning: Don't attempt this trip immediately after heavy rains; Big Tujunga turns into a raging torrent and has claimed several lives in recent years.

Description

Drive up the Angeles Crest Highway to Clear Creek Junction, and then left on the Angeles Forest Highway (County Road N3) to an unmarked parking area shaded by a lone incense cedar on your right, 15.5 miles from La Cañada. If you reach the Narrows Bridge, you've driven 0.3 mile too far. Be sure to display your Adventure Pass on your parked vehicle.

Cross the highway and follow an unmarked trail steeply down the slope. Halfway down, the trail divides into several very steep paths. Take extreme care as you descend the last 100 feet to the canyon floor. Please do not climb down over the concrete gauging station. Here, in the middle of Big Tujunga Narrows, you have a choice.

If you decide to venture upstream, the first 0.75 mile is easygoing, as you pass the confluence of Mill Creek and walk under the spectacular Narrows Bridge, looming far above, a marvel of steel and concrete. Beyond the bridge, Big Tujunga twists and turns in an easterly direction, and you must scramble over and around jumbo streamside boulders. Notice the chaparral on the sun-drenched south-facing slope and the conifer forest on the shady north-facing slope—very characteristic of canyons in the San Gabriels. In 0.75 mile you reach a waterfall. This is as far as you can safely go, so return the same way.

If you choose to explore downstream from the Flood Control District gauging station, the going is more difficult. In 0.25 mile you reach the granite-enclosed gorge of the lower Narrows and its foot-wetting fords. It is 1.5 rough miles down to Forest Road 3N27, through an area of cascades and small waterfalls. This traverse is for experienced cross-country hikers only and should never be attempted during times of high water.

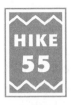

MOUNT GLEASON ROAD TO MOUNT GLEASON

HIKE LENGTH: 5 miles round-trip; 1,000' elevation gain
DIFFICULTY: Moderate
SEASON: May–October
TOPO MAP: *Acton*

Features

The long, forested hogback of Mount Gleason (6,502') dominates the western end of the San Gabriels. From Gleason's broad summit you look north across the drab expanse of the Mojave Desert, and on the clearest of days, you can just make out, far on the distant horizon, the angular snow-streaked peaks of the southern High Sierra.

The mountain is drenched in history. In 1869 George Gleason, first postmaster of Ravenna and superintendent of the rich Eureka Mine near present-day Acton, climbed the north slope in quest of the timber stands he saw on top. Instead, he found gold. Men swarmed up the mountain, and the Mount Gleason Mining District was organized. Transporting the gold-bearing quartz down the steep slopes to the mill in Soledad Canyon was a harrowing process. Logs were fastened behind the ore-filled wagons, pulled by eight-mule teams, to slow the descent. Even so, accidents occurred with regularity. The most active period for the Gleason Mines was 1888–1896, when some 20 prospects were being worked and a five-stamp mill was erected high on the north slope. The richest mines were named the Gleason, the Lost Padres, and the Eagle. There has been no activity in recent years, and only the miners' ghosts remain now.

This once was a delightful stroll through forest and chaparral, on trail all the way, with far-ranging desert views. The 2009 Station Fire changed all that when it roared through here, claiming the lives of two firefighters and incinerating most of the forest. The shady pine and fir groves that dotted the higher slopes are now mostly charred stumps. It will take many decades for the mountain to regain its old beauty.

Description

Drive up the Angeles Crest Highway to Clear Creek Junction, and then left on the Angeles Forest Highway (County Road N3) to Mill Creek Summit, 23 miles from La Cañada. Turn left (west) and follow Mount Gleason Road (signed MESSENGER FLATS *12*), passing a

Pacific Crest Trail junction in 2.5 miles (you can start your hike here if you don't mind adding 8 miles round-trip to it), to a road junction in 6 miles, just outside the site of a Youth Conservation Camp that was destroyed in the 2009 fire. Drive left and continue on Mount Gleason Road 0.5 mile to where it bottoms out. Park in the clearing to your right. Be sure to display your Adventure Pass on your parked vehicle. *Note:* The gate to Mount Gleason Road is sometimes closed at Angeles Forest Highway. Check ahead with the US Forest Service to ensure that it's open before attempting this hike.

Walk right to the lower, east end of the clearing, where you will see a yellow locked gate and a poor dirt road descending northward. Pass the gate and walk down the road about 25 yards, to where you intersect the Pacific Crest Trail. Go left and follow the PCT as it climbs west, and then northwest. You cross an old dirt road and, 0.25 mile farther, make a sharp switchback up to the top of Mount Gleason's west ridge. Leave the PCT here and go left (east) over several hummocks to the top. A few hardy pines somehow survived the ravages of fire, but mostly, you're in a tree graveyard. The large concrete structure you see here is the foundation of a disassembled Air Force radar dome.

When you've seen enough, return the way you came.

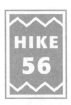

MILL CREEK SUMMIT
TO MT. PACIFICO CAMPGROUND

HIKE LENGTH: 6 miles one way; 2,200' elevation gain
DIFFICULTY: Moderate
SEASON: May–October
TOPO MAP: *Pacifico Mountain*

Features

Note: The route described here, along the Pacific Crest Trail, is currently—as of spring 2013—closed due to the 2009 Station Fire. Check ahead with the US Forest Service to determine if it has been reopened. Mount Pacifico can still be reached via Forest Road 3N17 from Mill Creek Summit, 6 miles one way. This route lies along the southern slope of the mountain, is shadeless until you near Mount Pacifico, and is not nearly as attractive as the PCT route. Forest Road 3N17 is currently closed to vehicular traffic. Also note that although the mountaintop and campground area was spared from heavy damage by the fire, as of this writing, the campground remains closed.

Pacifico Mountain looms high on the northern rampart of the San Gabriels, offering far-reaching panoramas over Antelope Valley and the Mojave Desert. On days when the sky is clear of the usual desert haze, the viewer can make out, on the distant horizon, the sawtooth peaks of the High Sierra and the distinct cone-shaped summit of Telescope Peak overlooking Death Valley.

Legend says that 7,124-foot Pacifico Mountain and its all-year spring were a hangout of Tiburcio Vásquez and his gang of horse thieves in the 1870s. In fact, the infamous bandido supposedly gave it the name Pacifico because he could see the Pacific Ocean from the top.

This very pleasant, view-rich trip follows the easy-graded Pacific Crest Trail most of the way, and then climbs to the Mt. Pacifico Campground, right on the summit, via the campground road or the west ridge. If you reverse the trip, it's all downhill. A car shuttle is recommended.

Description

Drive up the Angeles Crest Highway to Clear Creek Junction, and then left on the Angeles Forest Highway (L.A. County Road N3) to Mill Creek Summit, 23 miles from La Cañada. Drive another car to Mt. Pacifico Campground or arrange to be picked up at this spot. To

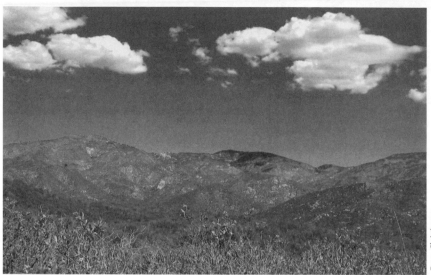

Pacifico Mountain

reach the latter from Mill Creek Summit, turn right (east) and follow Forest Road 3N17 to the summit campground, 6 miles. Be sure to display your Adventure Pass on your parked vehicle.

From the Mill Creek Summit parking area, cross Forest Road 3N17 to the signed Pacific Crest Trail heading northeast. The trail climbs, and then contours just below and behind the US Forest Service maintenance station. Beyond, the pathway gently climbs eastward, then northward, through an open forest of big-cone Douglas-firs and interior live oaks, around the head of Tie Canyon. You ascend chaparral-clad slopes to a ridge crest, where expansive views open northward across Antelope Valley and the Mojave Desert. Then you round the ridge and turn south, intersecting an old, abandoned dirt road. Your trail follows the roadbed for 0.5 mile, and then turns left and ascends eastward, then southeast, under a cool canopy of oaks and Jeffrey pines. You reach a forested gap and a junction with the Mt. Pacifico Campground road in 5 miles. The Pacific Crest Trail, which you have been following, turns north, but you leave it here and have a choice of routes. You can follow the gently graded campground road to the summit, 1.25 miles, or climb the shorter but steeper west ridge to the top.

For a much easier trip, reverse it. Leave the Mt. Pacifico Campground road where it intersects the PCT, 0.25 mile up from Forest Road 3N17, and walk downhill all the way to Mill Creek Summit.

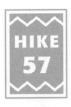

CHILAO TO DEVIL'S CANYON, SAN GABRIEL WILDERNESS

HIKE LENGTH: 7 miles round-trip; 1,500' elevation loss and gain
DIFFICULTY: Moderate
SEASON: November–April
TOPO MAPS: *Chilao Flat, Waterman Mountain*

Features

Fewer than 20 air miles from downtown Los Angeles is the San Gabriel Wilderness, 36,000 acres of rugged ridge and canyon country forever protected and preserved in its natural state. No roads, no resorts, and no noisy public campgrounds are here, only the primeval sounds of earth—the wind rustling leaves of pines and alders, the stream dancing over boulders and cascades, the wren-tit's staccato call, and, on rare occasions, the mountain lion darting through brush. Only three maintained trails enter this wilderness. Perhaps the most delightful one leaves the Angeles Crest at Chilao and descends steep slopes of chaparral, firs, and pines into the shaded bowels of Devil's Canyon. Here, under a green canopy of alders and willows, alongside deep pools and miniature waterfalls, the hiker can find solitude on a day's outing or overnight backpack, and relive a part of the mountains as they once were.

The canyon lies along the eastern limit of the 2009 Station Fire burn area and did not suffer the kind of complete destruction that befell parts of the Big Tujunga watershed just west of here. You will pass through portions of burn area and then sections where the forest is mostly intact. The canyon bottom, along the stream, remains a shady oasis, a place to rest, contemplate, and meditate. Take care; this is an "upside-down" trip—downhill all the way in, uphill on the return. Many an out-of-condition rambler has stridden gaily down, only to labor painfully every upward step out.

Description

A prominent sign marks the Devil's Canyon trailhead on the Angeles Crest Highway, 27 miles from La Cañada and about 200 yards *before* you reach the Chilao Visitor Center turnoff. Leave your car in the large parking area on the left (west) side of the road, directly across

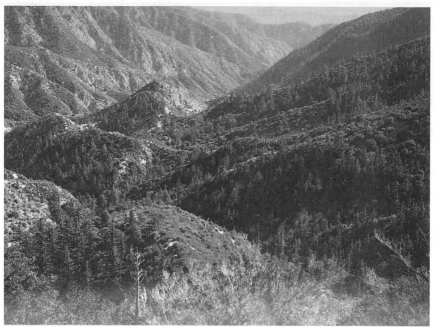

Devil's Canyon, San Gabriel Wilderness

from the trailhead. Be sure to display your Adventure Pass on your parked vehicle.

The trail, well maintained by the US Forest Service, is easy to follow although in somewhat rougher condition since the fire. It loses no time in descending the steep hillsides, alternately through stands of big-cone Douglas-firs on shady north faces and dense chaparral on sunnier slopes. You will see ample evidence of the Station Fire as you descend. About halfway down, the trail meets a small tributary creek and then follows it to the main canyon. At its end, on a shaded bench on your right, well above the stream, is a wilderness camping area.

It is possible, without inordinate difficulty for the average hiker, to follow Devil's Canyon downstream about 2 miles—crossing and recrossing the creek, boulder-hopping, and occasionally thrashing through willow and brush. Beyond this, the canyon narrows, sidewalls steepen, and waterfalls assume grander proportions: this is experts' country, only for the experienced climber with rope and climbing hardware.

Allow plenty of time for the return trip—at least twice than what it took to get in. Remember, it's all uphill.

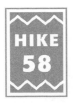

CHILAO TO HORSE FLATS, MOUNT HILLYER

HIKE LENGTH: 6 miles round-trip; 1,000' elevation gain
DIFFICULTY: Moderate
SEASON: All year
TOPO MAP: *Chilao Flat*

Features

The Chilao–Horse Flats country is a gentle region of rounded ridgetops, shallow draws, and small flats set deep in the heart of the San Gabriels. The forest here is open and parklike; tall Jeffrey pines and incense cedars cluster in sheltered recesses and dot the rolling hillsides. The chaparral is rich and green and the sky is a deep blue, with seldom a trace of the brown murkiness that so often invades the south slope of the range. And thankfully, there is comparatively little fire damage; the 2009 Station Fire was a near miss here. This is ideal picnicking, camping, and hiking country.

A century ago this was bandido country. The notorious Tiburcio Vásquez and his gang of horse thieves utilized Chilao and Horse Flats—then deep in the wilderness and little known—as refuges from the law, as hideouts where they could rest and plan their next raid, and as pastures for stolen horses. The great boulders of nearby Mount Hillyer furnished an impregnable fortress if pursuing posses came too close. One of Vásquez's men at Chilao was a herder named Jose Gonzales, noted among his cohorts for his skill with a knife. On one occasion he killed a bear with some slick knife work, earning the nickname Chillia ("hot stuff"). From this allegedly came the name Chilao.

There are no bandidos here now, and roads lace the region, but the country still holds appeal. This very pleasant trail hike takes you through the best of the Chilao–Horse Flats area, and it climbs through magnificent stands of Jeffrey pines and around jumbo boulders to the summit of Mount Hillyer.

Description

Drive up the Angeles Crest Highway to the turnoff for the Chilao Visitor Center (closed as of this writing), 27 miles from La Cañada. Turn left and drive down the paved road, passing the visitor center, 0.5 mile to a clearing on your right, where a sign indicates SILVER MOCCASIN TRAIL. Park here. (This road is closed November 16–March 31; you will have to park along Angeles Crest Highway and walk in, adding 1 mile to the round-trip distance.) Be sure to display your Adventure Pass on your parked vehicle.

Proceed 1 mile up the trail as it switchbacks through chaparral and clusters of Jeffrey pines—the 2009 Station Fire did some damage here—to a junction just short of Horse Flats Campground. Turn left, leaving the Silver Moccasin Trail, and follow the path 100 yards to the south edge of the campground. A sign to your left indicates MT. HILLYER, 2 MILES. Proceed up the Mount Hillyer Trail through open clusters of manzanitas, scrub oaks, and Jeffrey pines and around a maze of giant granite boulders, to the broad summit of Mount Hillyer. You can't see much from the forested top, but if you walk several hundred feet southwest onto the firebreak, you are rewarded with a fine panorama of the rolling bandido country to the south and southeast, and the broad trench of fire-scorched Alder Creek dropping off to the west.

Return the same way. One very pleasant option, adding 2 miles to the round-trip, is to go north from the summit along the ridgetop trail, which climbs gently over two nubbins before descending to a junction with the Santa Clara Divide Road (3N17). Turn right (southeast) and follow the paved road, and then right again on the Horse Flats Campground access road to Horse Flats, where you meet your trail of ascent. From here, follow the same route down to your car.

A very easy way to climb Mount Hillyer is from the Santa Clara Divide Road (3N17) mentioned above.

Drive the Angeles Crest Highway to its junction with the Santa Clara Divide Road, indicated by a metal sign, 29.5 miles from La Cañada and 1.5 miles past Chilao. Turn left (west) and follow the paved road past the entrance to Horse Flats Campground to a saddle where the road crosses a crest, 3 miles from the highway and 0.3 mile beyond the campground entrance. Park in the parking area to your left.

Walk south along the divide (once a dirt road), and then up the broad fuel break, over several nubbins to the unmarked summit, 1.25 miles.

You can cut 2 miles off the round-trip by driving to Horse Flats Campground. Turn left off Angeles Crest Highway 2.5 miles north of Chilao, where a sign indicates SANTA CLARA DIVIDE ROAD, and proceed 2.5 miles on this road to the campground.

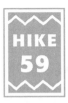

THREE POINTS TO TWIN PEAKS SADDLE, SAN GABRIEL WILDERNESS, TWIN PEAKS, MOUNT WATERMAN, AND BUCKHORN

HIKE LENGTH: 14 miles (total); 3,700' elevation gain
DIFFICULTY: Strenuous
SEASON: June–October
TOPO MAP: *Waterman Mountain*

Features

This trip traverses the high country along the northern boundary of the San Gabriel Wilderness and climbs the two major peaks in the region. From the ramparts of Mount Waterman and Twin Peaks (especially the latter), you look down over the extremely rugged upper reaches of Devil's and Bear Canyons, the wildest mountain country in the San Gabriels. Here, among the crags and in the deep recesses, are the undisturbed lairs of mountain lions, black bears, and

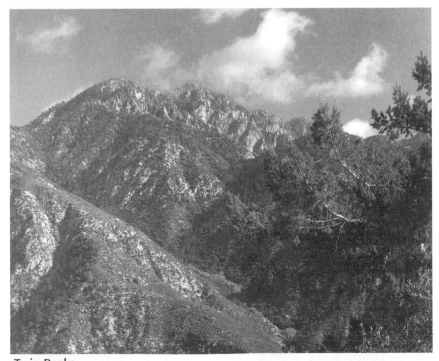

Twin Peaks

bighorn sheep, animals seldom seen in the more frequented parts of the range.

This is delightful wilderness country. The topography is more broken than in most other parts of the range, and jumbo boulders dot the slopes. The chaparral is tall and richly textured. The forest, primarily Jeffrey and ponderosa pines, is open and parklike, carpeted with pine needles. Near Twin Peaks Saddle are some of the most beautiful stands of incense cedars in the range. On sunny slopes, lupines stand bright and pagodalike in early summer. Half a dozen trickling rills line the route during early season, only to disappear one by one as the dry months progress.

A car shuttle between Three Points and Buckhorn is required if you wish to do the full traverse. Although the total trip is classified as strenuous, parts of it can be taken and thoroughly enjoyed by the neophyte. A 2-mile stroll up-trail from Three Points will reward the beginner with superb vistas into Devil's Canyon. If you are a hiker of moderate ability, you can continue 4 more miles to Twin Peaks Saddle and return. This high wilderness is really too good to be reserved for only the strongest; it is there for all.

Description

Drive the Angeles Crest Highway to Three Points junction, 2.4 miles beyond (north of) Chilao, near highway mileage marker 52.60. Turn left on Santa Clara Divide Road (sign says HORSE FLATS 2) and follow the dirt road about 100 yards to a paved parking area on your left. If you're doing the full traverse, shuttle another car to the parking area just before the road to Buckhorn Campground, 5 miles farther on the Angeles Crest. Be sure to display your Adventure Pass on your parked vehicles.

From the parking area just above Three Points, take the trail that leads down to the Pacific Crest Trail, 50 yards. Turn left and follow the PCT down to the highway, which must be crossed with care (on weekends some vehicles and motorcycles use the Angeles Crest as a speedway). Pick up the PCT on the east side of the highway, which is marked by a large wooden sign indicating, among other things, MT. WATERMAN, 7 MILES. The PCT begins climbing above the highway; in about 100 yards you reach a junction. Here, you go right (sign says MT. WATERMAN) and leave the PCT. Your trail starts zigzagging up the west spine of the mountain. There is evidence of the 2009 Station Fire here—the eastern edge of the burn area. After gaining about

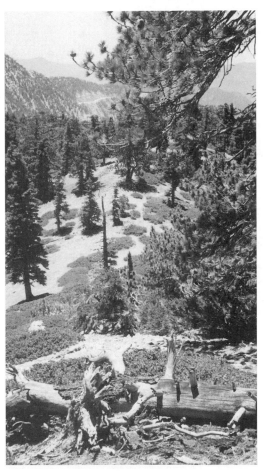

Mount Waterman east ridge

600 feet the route levels off and traverses around the long, indented slopes of Waterman. The deep trench of Devil's Canyon is constantly in view to your right. Keep a sharp lookout for bighorn sheep; they are occasionally seen here. The trail rounds the mountain and after 5 miles reaches a junction—left up to Mount Waterman, right down to Twin Peaks Saddle. Go right, and follow the trail 1 mile, descending 400 feet to Twin Peaks Saddle. Here, the maintained trail ends, but a pathway worn by climbers, very steep in places, leads up the north slope of Twin Peaks 1,200 feet to the summit (the eastern of the two peaks is higher). This is the climax of the trip; from the top you see nature's pattern of the entire San Gabriel Wilderness, a panorama you'll find nowhere else.

Return to Twin Peaks Saddle, and then walk up-trail 1 mile to the aforementioned junction. This time, take the right fork and climb 1,200 feet more (2 miles) to the summit of Mount Waterman, the highest point in the wilderness area. After taking in the view (excellent but not as good as from Twin Peaks), descend the main trail to Buckhorn (*see* Hike 60).

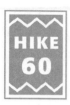

BUCKHORN TO MOUNT WATERMAN

HIKE 60

HIKE LENGTH: 6 miles round-trip; 1,300' elevation gain
DIFFICULTY: Moderate
SEASON: June–October
TOPO MAP: *Waterman Mountain*

Features

The San Gabriels were almost totally wild and unexplored, and grizzlies frequented the area when, in 1889, Bob Waterman; his bride, Liz; and Commodore Ferry Switzer—all of famed Switzer's Camp in the Arroyo Seco—made a three-week trip across the range to the desert and back. En route they scrambled up the highest mountain in the vicinity to get their bearings. On the summit they built a cairn and left a register. In honor of Liz, who they believed to be the first white woman to cross the range, the two men christened the peak Lady Waterman Mountain. Years later, when the U.S. Geological Survey mapped the mountain, it left off the Lady part of the designation. Bob Waterman, who lived many years longer in Pasadena, tried several times to restore his wife's honor by putting the Lady back on the peak but to no avail. Today it's just Mount Waterman.

Mount Waterman, at 8,038 feet, is best known to skiers. Several ski lifts ascend the broad north slope of the mountain, making it one of the most popular winter sports areas in the range. But in summer, when the snow is gone, Mount Waterman becomes the sole domain of the hiker. Most climbers take this well-graded, easy-to-follow trail from Buckhorn, the shortest way up the mountain.

Waterman is an elongated, broad-summited mountain, shaped like a mammoth "U," with three high points. The highest of the high points lies near the southwestern edge of the summit plateau. From here, you are rewarded with a panoramic vista of the entire western San Gabriels, with particularly fine views into the depths of Devil's Canyon.

Description

Drive the Angeles Crest Highway to a point near highway mileage marker 58.0, 34 miles from La Cañada. Park on one of the wide shoulders alongside the highway. Be sure to display your Adventure Pass on your parked vehicle.

The trailhead here is confusing because of a profusion of fire roads and footpaths that climb the north slope of Mount Waterman from the highway. The correct trail is the one farthest to the left (east). At the SAN GABRIEL WILDERNESS sign, walk about 30 feet up the fire road, and then go left on a section of trail that parallels the highway for a short distance, crosses another fire road, and begins to ascend the forested slope. After climbing southward through tall stands of Jeffrey pines and incense cedars for 1.25 miles, the trail reaches a saddle on Waterman's east ridge; from here you look

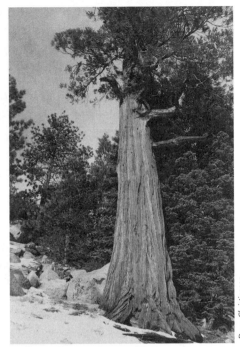

Jeffrey pine on Mount Waterman

Doug Christiansen

down into the wild upper reaches of Bear Canyon and to Twin Peaks beyond. The trail now turns west and climbs to a junction with the Twin Peaks Trail, 0.5 mile. Go right and continue up to the broad, undulating summit plateau. The trail does not reach the actual summit of Waterman; when it turns northwest and begins to descend, leave the trail and head southwest, past a subsidiary summit, about 500 yards to the true summit.

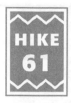

CLOUDBURST SUMMIT TO COOPER CANYON, COOPER CANYON TRAIL CAMP, PLEASANT VIEW RIDGE WILDERNESS, BUCKHORN CAMPGROUND

HIKE 61

HIKE LENGTH: 6 miles round-trip;
1,300' elevation loss, 800' elevation gain
DIFFICULTY: Moderate
SEASON: May–October
TOPO MAP: *Waterman Mountain*

Features

Beautiful, woodsy Cooper Canyon, a major tributary of Little Rock Creek, has long been a favorite of hikers. Its little singing creek, shaded by beautiful stands of Jeffrey and sugar pines, cedars, alders, and oaks, was once a favorite American Indian haunt. According to mountain historian Will Thrall, braves camped at Buckhorn, just over the ridge, and sent their women and children here while the men hunted and raised a ruckus. For many years the old American Indian campsite in the upper canyon, now Cooper Canyon Trail Camp, was known as Squaw Camp. The canyon became the favorite hunting ground of Pasadena brothers Ike and Tom Cooper during the 1890s, when deer and bear were plentiful. The Cooper brothers are long gone, but their exploits are eternalized by the canyon name.

Part of this scenic hike lies within the new Pleasant View Ridge Wilderness, 26,752 acres set aside by Congress in 2009. No permit is required to enter.

This loop trip, requiring a car shuttle between Cloudburst Summit on the Angeles Crest Highway and Buckhorn Campground, takes you down through this richly forested recess where nature's stillness reigns supreme. To make the trip more leisurely and allow time to enjoy the beauty of this canyon country, stay overnight at Cooper Canyon Trail Camp.

Description

Drive up the Angeles Crest Highway to Cloudburst Summit, 33 miles from La Cañada. Park in the clearing to the left (north) of the highway, where the fire road descends into Cooper Canyon, taking care not to block the dirt roadway. The trip will finish at Buckhorn Campground, 1.5 miles east, just off the highway. Note

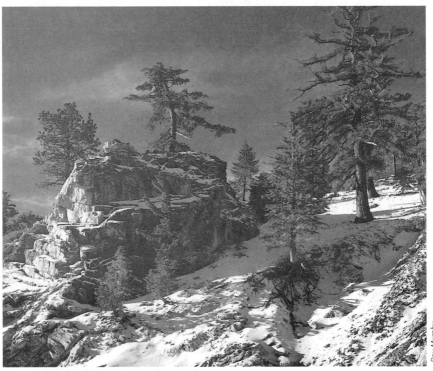

San Gabriels high country after spring storm

that the campground is closed in winter; during this season (not recommended unless you're experienced in and equipped for snow hiking) you will need to leave your second car along the highway outside Buckhorn, adding another 0.75 mile and 200 feet to the total distance and elevation gain required to reach your car. If you plan to walk back up the highway to Cloudburst Summit, it's a total of 2.25 extra miles. Be certain to display your Adventure Pass on your parked vehicles.

Proceed past the locked gate and 1.75 miles down the fire road to Cooper Canyon Trail Camp, on a forested bench to your right. Tables, stoves, and toilet facilities make this a convenient overnight camping spot. Take the broad trail (formerly a road) down Cooper Canyon 1.25 miles to its junction with the Burkhart Trail leading up to Buckhorn. Turn right and follow the latter 1.75 miles up to the Buckhorn Campground hiker's parking area (*see* Hike 62).

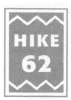

BUCKHORN CAMPGROUND TO COOPER CANYON, PLEASANT VIEW RIDGE WILDERNESS, LITTLE ROCK CREEK

HIKE LENGTH: 5 miles round-trip; 900' elevation loss and gain
DIFFICULTY: Moderate
SEASON: May–October
TOPO MAP: *Waterman Mountain*

Features

Nestled in deep canyons north of Mount Waterman and Kratka Ridge are woodsy hideaways where nature, at her quiet, pristine best, still reigns relatively undisturbed by the markings of man. Buckhorn Canyon, Cooper Canyon, and Upper Little Rock Creek are three of the most delightful sylvan recesses in Angeles National Forest. Sparkling streams glide, dance, and tumble over boulders and cascade down miniature waterfalls, shaded by a magnificent forest of Jeffrey pines, sugar pines, incense cedars, alders, and oaks. Ferns and lush grasses sprout emerald-green along the banks, and in spring and early summer, mountain wildflowers add a dash of color.

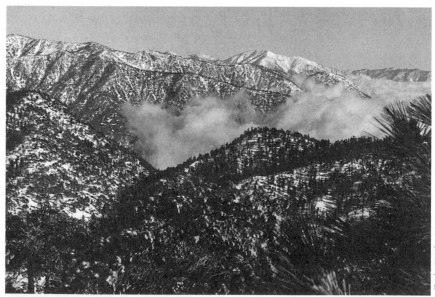

Charles Kassler

East from Pleasant View Ridge

This trip—one of the best in the San Gabriels—takes you from Buckhorn Public Campground down along the slopes of Buckhorn Canyon into shady Cooper Canyon and on to Little Rock Creek. Anglers as well as nature lovers will enjoy the jaunt, for there are rainbow trout in Little Rock Creek. You're in the new Pleasant View Ridge Wilderness, created in 2009, 26,752 acres forever set aside to remain in their natural state (no permit is required to enter).

Pine- and cedar-shaded Buckhorn was once an American Indian haunt, back when Shoshonean peoples frequented the range in search of acorns, pine nuts, and wild game. You can still find large boulders with mortar holes worn into them, used by American Indians to grind meal. After the American Indian came the white hunter. Buckhorn was a backcountry hangout for hunters, seeking the abundant wild game. The name Buckhorn dates from this period—a pair of king-size buckhorns was once nailed to a tree here. Today Buckhorn is a well-equipped public campground; recently renovated, it is a favorite of Angeles National Forest campers.

Description
Drive up the Angeles Crest Highway to Buckhorn Campground, 34 miles from La Cañada and 0.5 mile past the Mount Waterman Ski Area. Turn left and follow the Buckhorn Campground Road through the campground to the hikers' parking area just beyond. (Do not park in the campground proper.) Be sure to display your Adventure Pass on your parked vehicle. If it's winter and the campground is closed, you will have to park along the highway and walk in to the trailhead, an extra 0.75 mile each way.

Take the Burkhart Trail from the north end of the parking area down-canyon along the left (northeast) slope. Follow this trail as it descends through pines and cedars into Cooper Canyon, where you intersect the Cooper Canyon Trail (*see* Hike 61), 1.75 miles. Take the right fork and follow the trail 0.25 mile down Cooper Canyon, through a wilderness garden of green around small Cooper Canyon Falls, to Little Rock Creek. Here, Burkhart Trail intersects the Rattlesnake Trail leading east up Little Rock Creek to the Angeles Crest Highway (*see* Hike 64).

There is no trail down Little Rock Creek; however, you can explore the canyon quite a distance by boulder-hopping. Take care if it's spring and the snowpack on the higher mountains is melting; Little Rock Creek runs high then.

Return the way you came—all uphill now.

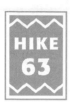

BUCKHORN TO PLEASANT VIEW RIDGE
WILDERNESS, LITTLE ROCK CREEK, BURKHART SADDLE, PLEASANT VIEW RIDGE

HIKE 63

HIKE LENGTH: 14 miles round-trip; 3,300' elevation gain
DIFFICULTY: Strenuous
SEASON: May–October
TOPO MAPS: *Waterman Mountain, Juniper Hills*

Features

Long, sinuous Pleasant View Ridge lives up to its name. A hiker resting in the shade of tall Jeffrey pines on its crest can gaze far out into the seemingly endless Mojave Desert. On the clearest of days, you can make out the tawny, sharp-toothed ramparts of the southern Sierra Nevada more than 60 miles in the distance. The area was designated as wilderness in 2009, 26,752 acres forever preserved in their natural, wild state (a permit is not required to enter).

Looking at Pleasant View Ridge from the Angeles Crest Highway, you may think that it is close at hand. But it's farther than you realize. Separating the ridge from the main body of the range is the V-shaped trench of Little Rock Creek, a desert-bound creek whose canyon holds sylvan surprises where you might least expect to find them. To reach Pleasant View, you must descend into the deep canyon and climb up the other side.

Be in shape for this one. It's up and down both ways, with little level going. If the day is warm, carry plenty of water.

Description

Drive up the Angeles Crest Highway to the Buckhorn Campground hikers' parking area (*see* Hike 62), 34 miles from La Cañada. Be sure to display your Adventure Pass on your parked vehicle. If it's winter—recommended only for those experienced in snow hiking—and the gate on the campground road is closed, you will need to park along the highway, adding 0.75 mile each way to the total.

Walk down the rear access road into the campground and turn right. Follow the trail that leaves from near the east end of the campground and descends to Little Rock Creek, 2 miles (*see* Hike 62 for trail description). Here, you intersect the Rattlesnake Trail coming down from Eagles Roost Picnic Area (*see* Hike 64). Take the left fork and follow the Burkhart Trail as it steadily climbs around a ridge, crosses a small creek (which has water in spring and early summer), and zigzags 3.5 miles up 1,300 feet to Burkhart Saddle.

Here, you have three options:

1. You can enjoy the desert view from here and return the way you came.

2. You can turn left (west) and follow an unmarked trail up around the slopes of Will Thrall Peak to a pleasant, Jeffrey-forested bench just west of the high point, and then scramble up to the 7,983-foot summit of Pleasant View Ridge, slightly more than a mile, with a 1,000-foot elevation gain from the saddle. From here the view is outstanding.

3. You can descend the desert side of the Burkhart Trail to Devil's Punchbowl (*see* Hike 67), if you can arrange a very long car shuttle.

Whichever option you take, you are certain to enjoy this northern extremity of the San Gabriels, where the aroma of desert sage blends with the sweet scent of mountain pines and cedars.

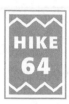

EAGLES ROOST PICNIC AREA TO LITTLE ROCK CREEK, PLEASANT VIEW RIDGE WILDERNESS

HIKE 64

HIKE LENGTH: 6 miles round-trip;
1,100' elevation gain and loss
DIFFICULTY: Moderate
SEASON: May–October
TOPO MAP: *Waterman Mountain*

Features

Note: The US Forest Service has temporarily—at least through spring 2013—closed the portion of Little Rock Creek described in this trip, to protect the habitat of the endangered mountain yellow-legged frog. Check with the US Forest Service before attempting this trip.

Some of the most magnificent canyon country in the San Gabriel Mountains lies on the desert slopes of the range. Nowhere is this more evident than in the uppermost reaches of Little Rock Creek, close under Kratka Ridge and Mount Williamson's southwest shoulder. The terrain is rugged and colorful—sheer crags of whitish rock stand in stark contrast to wrinkled slopes of reddish-brown and gray. Jeffrey, sugar, and Coulter pines, as well as white firs, incense cedars, and oaks, crowd canyon recesses and dot open ridges. The delightful stream, fed by springs high in the granite folds of Mount Williamson, runs all year.

This trip leaves the Angeles Crest Highway opposite Eagles Roost Picnic Area and descends the old Rattlesnake Trail (not as ominous as it sounds) into the upper reaches of Little Rock Creek. Once you leave the highway, you drop into recesses as magnificently wild as any in the range. If you like primitive canyon country relatively undisturbed by civilization, this hike should be a rewarding experience. The entire surrounding area north of the highway was officially declared a wilderness area in 2009.

Description

Drive up the Angeles Crest Highway to Eagles Roost Picnic Area, just before you reach a highway-maintenance shed, 39 miles from La Cañada. Park in the clearing. Be sure to display your Adventure Pass on your parked vehicle.

Cross the highway and descend west on the unmarked fire road into the head of Little Rock Creek. After 0.5 mile the fire road narrows into a regular trail, and then continues dropping to the canyon bottom, 0.5 mile farther. Here, amid a darkened forest and alongside the cold waters of the creek, you will be tempted to pause. A 200-yard side trip upstream brings you to a sparkling pool beneath a miniature waterfall. Back on the main route, follow the trail as it contours along the north slope of the gorge, heading downstream (west). For the next 2 miles, you round rocky points, with the creek far below, and pass through sheltered recesses. Finally, you drop down alongside the creek and reach a junction with the Burkhart Trail.

Here, you have several options. You can return up the Rattlesnake Trail, the way you came. You can turn left (southwest) and ascend the trail to Buckhorn Campground (*see* Hike 62). This makes a very pleasant circle trip and requires a 4-mile car shuttle between Eagles Roost and Buckhorn. Or you can turn right (north) and ascend the Burkhart Trail to Pleasant View Ridge (*see* Hike 63), and then return.

Experienced hikers have descended trailless Little Rock Creek from the Burkhart Trail all the way to the lower Little Rock Creek Road, 8 boulder-hopping miles. Heed two warnings if you want to try this: don't do it alone, and don't do it when the stream is high.

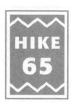

PLEASANT VIEW RIDGE WILDERNESS, MOUNT WILLIAMSON FROM ANGELES CREST HIGHWAY

HIKE LENGTH: 5 miles round-trip; 1,600' elevation gain
DIFFICULTY: Moderate
SEASON: June–October
TOPO MAP: *Crystal Lake*

Features

Mount Williamson, all 8,214 feet of it, stands tall and massive, jutting northward from the main crest of the range like a bold sentinel guarding the green high country from the withering influence of the desert 5,000 feet below. It is buttressed on the south by formidable cliffs, through which the Angeles Crest Highway tunnels, and on the north it plunges abruptly down to that fantastic jumble of whitish rocks known as the Devil's Punchbowl.

The mountain is named for Lieutenant Robert Stockton Williamson of the US Army, who led a reconnaissance of the north slopes of the San Gabriels for the Pacific Railroad Survey in 1853. He was looking for a railway route across the mountains. (Williamson didn't fail. He located *two* railway routes across the mountains—Soledad Pass and Cajon Pass.) The report he submitted to Congress contained the first detailed description of the desert side of the range.

From the summit of Mount Williamson, you get an eagle's-eye view of the broken country explored by this Army officer more than a century ago. It has changed much, but the strange geological features—the scarps, beeline valleys, troughs, sag ponds, and, most of all, the twisted and folded rocks of the Devil's Punchbowl—are the same. Mount Williamson towers directly above the San Andreas Rift Zone, the most monumental earthquake fault in the United States. Its unique pattern is readily observable to any who walk a short distance north from the summit and look down. The fault line can be seen extending along the entire northern base of the San Gabriels, from northwest to southeast. Only from Mount Williamson or from high points along Pleasant View Ridge, immediately to the northwest, do you get this perspective.

Description

You can start up Mount Williamson from either of two points along the Angeles Crest Highway, roughly 40 miles from La Cañada. One is an unnamed saddle 2.4 miles east of the old Kratka Ridge ski area,

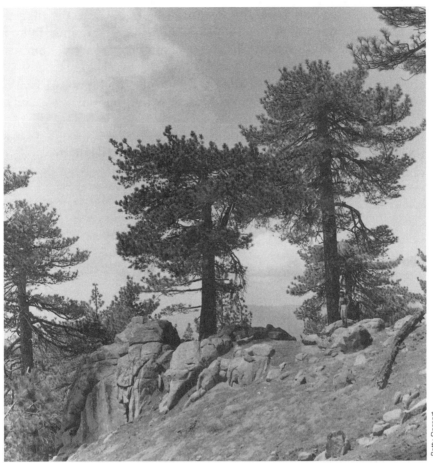

High on Mount Williamson Ridge

Betty Dessert

near highway mileage marker 62.50; the other is Islip Saddle, 1.6 miles farther east. From both places trails ascend to the south ridge of Williamson. If you can arrange a car shuttle, go up one way and down the other. Be sure to display your Adventure Pass on your parked vehicles. Although you're in the newly created Pleasant View Ridge Wilderness, no permit is needed.

From the unnamed, unsigned saddle beyond Kratka Ridge, take the trail at the east end of the parking area that switchbacks up Williamson's southwest ridge. You pass through an open forest of Jeffrey and ponderosa pines, with white firs becoming more abundant as you near 8,000 feet. In about 2 miles you reach the ridgetop and meet the trail coming up from Islip Saddle. From this point you are rewarded with a superb view southward, directly into the rugged trench of Bear Canyon, 3,000 feet below. To reach the summit, follow a faint trail northward along the ridge, climbing over several bumps to the 8,214-foot-high point overlooking the desert. This point is shown as the summit on the topo map, although a bump 0.25 mile northwest is 30 feet higher and offers a better view of the Devil's Punchbowl country.

If you start from Islip Saddle, take the trail that leads northwest up the ridge. After slightly less than 2 miles of steady climbing, you reach the ridgetop and meet the above-described trail coming up from the west.

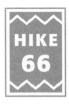

ANGELES CREST HIGHWAY TO PLEASANT VIEW RIDGE WILDERNESS, MOUNT WILLIAMSON, PLEASANT VIEW RIDGE, BURKHART SADDLE, LITTLE ROCK CREEK, EAGLES ROOST

HIKE 66

HIKE LENGTH: 12 miles round-trip; 3,500' elevation gain
DIFFICULTY: Strenuous
SEASON: June–October
TOPO MAPS: *Crystal Lake, Valyermo, Juniper Hills, Waterman Mountain*

Features

Note: The US Forest Service has temporarily—at least through spring 2013—closed the portion of this hike from Little Rock Creek to Eagles Roost to protect the habitat of the endangered mountain yellow-legged frog. Check with the US Forest Service before attempting this trip. An alternate route is described below.

This is a long up-and-down ramble over the northern crest of the San Gabriels, partly on trail, partly cross-country, through the newly created (in 2009) Pleasant View Ridge Wilderness (no permit required). The trip features a trailless traverse along the rim of Pleasant View Ridge between Mount Williamson and Burkhart Saddle, with continuous views over desert and high mountain country. It is a tough but rewarding experience for those in top physical condition. Don't try it alone; much of the terrain covered is seldom trod by human feet and rescue would be difficult. Carry all the water you need; most of the route is waterless.

Description

Drive up the Angeles Crest Highway to the beginning of the Mount Williamson west trail, 39 miles from La Cañada and 2.4 miles beyond the old Kratka Ridge ski area (*see* Hike 65). Be sure to display your Adventure Pass on your parked vehicle.

Take the trail to the summit of Mount Williamson (*see* Hike 65). Leave the trail at the summit and walk northwest along the top of Pleasant View Ridge, repeatedly losing and gaining several hundred feet of elevation, for 3 miles to Burkhart Saddle. This cross-country jaunt is open, through a rich forest of Jeffrey pines, but the steep up and down is tiring. Rest often and enjoy the superb desert view, with occasional glimpses down into the heart of the Devil's Punchbowl. From Burkhart Saddle, turn left (south) and follow the Burkhart

Trail down to Little Rock Creek (*see* Hike 63). From the creek, pick up the Rattlesnake Trail and follow it east, along the north slope of the canyon, up to the Angeles Crest Highway opposite Eagles Roost Picnic Area (*see* Hike 64). Walk northeast on the highway 0.5 mile to your car.

An alternative, if the Rattlesnake Trail is still off-limits, is to continue from where the Burkhart Trail meets Little Rock Creek, and follow the Burkhart Trail up to Buckhorn Campground (*see* Hike 63). This option requires a 6-mile car shuttle.

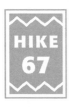

BURKHART TRAIL: DEVIL'S PUNCHBOWL TO PLEASANT VIEW RIDGE, PLEASANT VIEW RIDGE WILDERNESS

HIKE LENGTH: 10 miles round-trip; 2,300' elevation gain
DIFFICULTY: Moderate
SEASON: October–June
TOPO MAP: *Juniper Hills*

Features

South from Littlerock and Pearblossom, a number of rounded ridge-lines rise rather abruptly from the desert. Most prominent of these is Pleasant View Ridge, a long, sinuous hogback that begins its upward trend near Juniper Hills, leads southeasterly, and reaches its climax at 8,214-foot Mount Williamson. The ridge is aptly named. A hiker resting atop one of its many welts can look down upon little valleys and low foothills resplendent with the Mojave's best-known symbol—the beautiful Joshua tree, sharing the landscape with clusters of mesquite, purple sage, and yucca. In springtime, after abundant rain, the foothills are carpeted with colorful wildflowers. Sturdy junipers and piñons dot the higher slopes. And in the distance, beyond the strange beeline wrinkles of the San Andreas Fault, the Mojave Desert sprawls far and wide.

The Burkhart Trail, built years ago by a rancher of that name, is the only maintained footpath onto Pleasant View Ridge. The trail ascends the steep west slopes of Cruthers Creek from the desert to Burkhart Saddle, a distinct gap on the crest between Will Thrall Peak and Pallett Mountain. Except in a few places, it is gently graded as it climbs steadily from Joshua trees and sages through a piñon forest, and finally into Jeffrey pine country along the ridgetop.

The Burkhart Trail is a fitting introduction to the desert side of the San Gabriels, a side not well known to most Southern California hikers.

Description

Drive to Pearblossom on CA 138, and then south and southeast on County Road N6 to Devil's Punchbowl County Park, 8 miles. The park is open sunrise–sunset; parking is free.

To begin the hike, walk south from the nature center and pick up the trail as it passes behind the silver water tank and veers right at a junction signed BURKHART SADDLE 6.2 MILES. Follow the trail as it contours the mountain slope through Jeffrey pines and manzanitas. You drop into Cruthers Creek, and then climb the west slope and traverse upward high above the creek through piñons. You pass a small spring (which has water only in rainy season) and finally reach Burkhart Saddle, from where you look down into Little Rock Creek.

You now have several options. You can return to where you started. You can climb a faint trail leading right (west) up Pleasant View Ridge, around Will Thrall Peak, ending on a small flat on the crest (1.5 miles from the saddle). Or you can descend south from Burkhart Saddle into Little Rock Creek and on up to Buckhorn on the Angeles Crest Highway (*see* Hike 63). Another option is to continue east, on your return, via the new High Desert Trail across the top of Devil's Punchbowl to South Fork Campground (*see* Hike 69). Each of these options requires a car shuttle.

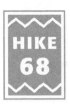

DEVIL'S PUNCHBOWL COUNTY PARK

HIKE LENGTH: 1-mile loop; 300' elevation gain and loss
DIFFICULTY: Easy
SEASON: October–June
TOPO MAP: *Valyermo*

Features

The great San Andreas Rift Zone cuts a beeline swath along the desert side of the San Gabriels. Many interesting geological features lie along this monumental earthquake fault system, but none so strange as the fantastic jumble of whitish rocks known as the Devil's Punchbowl. Within this mile-wide depression rise row upon row of weathered sandstone blocks, many of them tilted so as to resemble plates standing on edge, others folded and broken like huge slices of fancy pudding.

In 1963 this unique geological formation became a Los Angeles County park. A paved road was built on its western rim, and a wide, well-graded loop trail was hacked out down into the bowl.

Although only a short down-and-up walk, this otherworldly loop trip into the Devil's Punchbowl is one of the most interesting treks in the range. The trail passes beside weird sandstone outcrops, and at the bottom of the bowl, a playful stream cascades over, around, and through the slanted formations. Hardy piñons and manzanita thickets cling to precipitous footholds between the rocks.

Description

Drive to Pearblossom on CA 138, and then south and southeast on County Road N6 to Devil's Punchbowl County Park, 8 miles. The park is open sunrise–sunset; parking is free.

From the parking area, walk east past the park headquarters (which has restrooms, picnic tables, and interpretive displays) to the well-marked beginning of the trail. Follow the trail as it winds 300 feet down into the punchbowl, turns right just above the bottom, and then ascends back up to the parking area. The trail is gently graded for the most part (one short, steep pitch on the way out), and it is well worth the stride down and the huff-and-puff back out just to see first-hand what nature, in a fit of originality, has wrought.

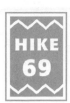

SOUTH FORK CAMPGROUND
TO DEVIL'S PUNCHBOWL

HIKE LENGTH: 6 miles round-trip; 1,000' elevation gain
DIFFICULTY: Moderate
SEASON: October–June
TOPO MAP: *Valyermo*

Features

This trip climbs over a ridge and enters the "back door" of the Devil's Punchbowl. It visits the wilder eastern part of the jumbled depression, a section not reached by the loop trail from county park headquarters (*see* Hike 68). It takes you to the strangest, most unique formation in the punchbowl—the huge white rock mass, sheer on three sides, known as the Devil's Chair. Those with vivid imaginations can make out the devil himself sitting on his throne, lording over his topsy-turvy domain.

You may wish to continue westward across the top of the punchbowl on the High Desert Trail, and then north on the Burkhart Trail connection to park headquarters. With a 6-mile car shuttle, you can hike clear across the park and see it all.

Description

From CA 138, turn south at Pearblossom onto Longview Road, and then left (southeast) on Valyermo Road past Valyermo, and right (south) on Big Rock Creek Road. Roughly 2.5 miles from this junction, turn south on a marked dirt road to South Fork Campground, 1 mile. Leave your car in the hikers' parking area, to your right about 100 yards before the campground. Be sure to display your Adventure Pass on your parked vehicle.

Walk south from the parking lot, pick up the trail, and follow it south about 50 yards to a junction, where you turn right (west), cross the boulder-strewn creek bed, and climb through piñons, scrub oaks, manzanitas, and mountain mahoganies to a saddle on the ridge. You contour, and then drop into Holcomb Canyon. Here, you find a rare meeting of three plant communities: pine, piñon-juniper, and streamside woodland. By late spring the yuccas are in full bloom. The trail fords tiny Holcomb Creek and then zigzags over another ridge, skirting the upper section of the devil's domain. You pass near the huge rock promontory known as the Devil's Chair, where a breathtaking

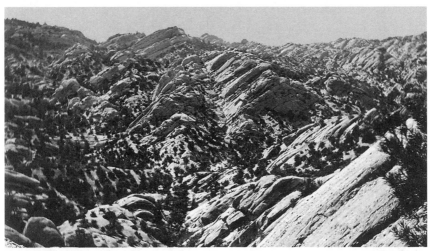

Will Thrall

Devil's Punchbowl

view of the punchbowl is obtained. If you venture onto the Devil's Chair, stay within the protective fence. You can explore other geological features above the punchbowl, but don't venture too close to cliffs or steep slopes. If you're not sure-footed, stay on the trail.

Return the way you came. A very attractive option is to continue west on the High Desert Trail, traversing the forest-clad slopes above the punchbowl, to the Burkhart Trail connection, and turn north on the latter down to park headquarters, 5.8 miles. You need a car shuttle for this (*see* Hike 67).

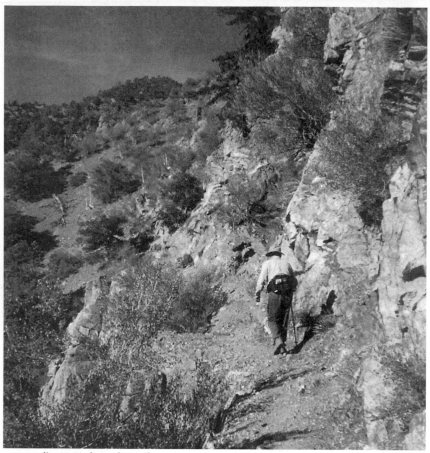

Ascending South Fork Trail

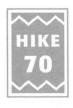

SOUTH FORK TRAIL: SOUTH FORK CAMPGROUND TO ISLIP SADDLE

HIKE 70

HIKE LENGTH: 10 miles round-trip; 2,100' elevation gain
DIFFICULTY: Moderate
SEASON: All year (upper part may be snowbound after winter storms)
TOPO MAPS: *Valyermo, Crystal Lake*

Features

The north front of the San Gabriel Mountains rises abruptly out of the desert, especially the parts north of the middle and eastern high country. Some of the canyons that incise this rampart are quite imposing, being deep, V-shaped gorges. Probably the most impressive of these north-facing canyons is the South Fork of Big Rock Creek, which carves a steep path as it drops from high on the Angeles Crest down into the San Andreas Rift region at the foot of the mountains.

An old trail—once a major route into the high country, before the Angeles Crest Highway forever changed the face of the mountains— climbs up-canyon all the way from South Fork Campground to Islip Saddle, passing from piñons to pines, from sages to snowbrushes, from cacti to buckthorns. The trail is seldom trod nowadays, for it culminates at that busy transmountain thoroughfare, the Angeles Crest Highway. But its lower and middle parts hold appeal—the foliage is a curious blend of desert and alpine, and the landscape is often more vertical than horizontal.

Description

From CA 138, turn south at Pearblossom onto Longview Road, and then left (southeast) on Valyermo Road past Valyermo, and right (south) on Big Rock Creek Road. Roughly 2.5 miles from this junction, turn south on a marked dirt road to South Fork Campground, 1 mile. Leave your car in the hikers' parking area, to your right about 100 yards before the campground. Be sure to display your Adventure Pass on your parked vehicle.

Walk south from the parking area on the well-marked trail, going left at a junction with the trail to Devil's Punchbowl, passing South Fork Campground on your left, and entering the deep canyon of Big Rock Creek's South Fork. Follow the trail up-canyon, through cottonwoods, oaks, maples, and alders, alongside the boulder-strewn streambed. After 0.25 mile the trail crosses to the west bank and begins climbing the canyon slopes, through scattered piñon pines. Piñons soon give way to Jeffrey pines as you climb higher, with the bubbling creek far down to your left. After about 4 miles, you pass the trickling Reed Spring, and then climb 1 more short mile to the parking area alongside the Angeles Crest Highway at Islip Saddle.

Return the way you came.

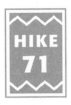

MANZANITA TRAIL: SOUTH FORK CAMPGROUND TO VINCENT GAP

HIKE 71

HIKE LENGTH: 11 miles round-trip; 2,400' elevation gain
DIFFICULTY: Moderate
SEASON: All year (upper part may be snowbound in winter)
Topo Maps: Valyermo, Mescal Creek

Features

The northern side of the San Gabriel Mountains differs markedly from the southern side that is more familiar to most hikers. The plant communities range from cottonwood-lined streams near the desert floor to forested canyon slopes covered with piñon pines, oaks, and manzanitas to the pine- and fir-forested peaks of the middle high country. Winter snows linger far longer on these north-facing, shady slopes than they do on the southern exposure visible from the Los Angeles area. Two huge tectonic plates, the Pacific Plate and the North American Plate, collide here, the incredible pressure forcing the mountains ever-higher and resulting in a variety of interesting geological features, most notably the strange, fantastic jumble of Devil's Punchbowl County Park (*see* Hikes 68 and 69).

This scenic trip follows the Punchbowl Fault, an inactive strand of the great San Andreas Fault, and passes through several areas where

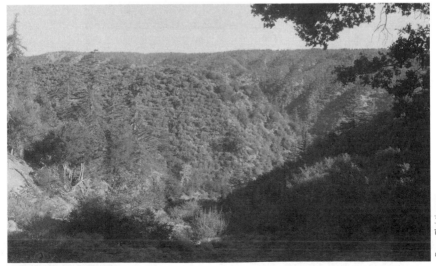

Big Rock Creek Canyon

Doug Christiansen

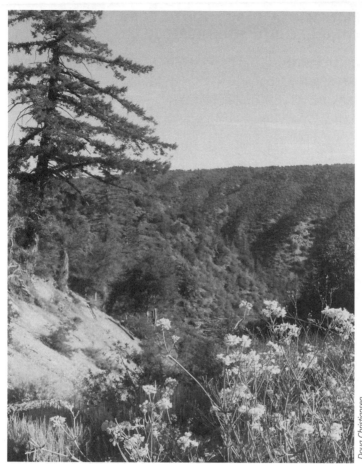

Along the Manzanita Trail

you can see the juxtaposition of different types of rock on either side of the fault trace. The trail, part of the High Desert National Recreation Trail, had fallen into a state of disrepair several years ago but has recently been reworked and put back in usable condition, thanks to the efforts of volunteers. It contours along the shady, north-facing slopes high above Big Rock Creek through a mixed forest of oaks, big-cone Douglas-firs, and, higher up, Jeffrey pines and white firs. It is a superb fall hike, when the air is cool and refreshing and the brilliant leaves of cottonwoods, maples, and black oaks provide a vivid contrast to the dull green and brown background. From the trail's end at Vincent Gap, a major junction, you have several options, described on the opposite page.

Description

From CA 138, turn south at Pearblossom onto Longview Road, and then left (southeast) on Valyermo Road past Valyermo, and right (south) on Big Rock Creek Road. Roughly 2.5 miles from this junction, turn south on a marked dirt road to South Fork Campground, 1 mile. Leave your car in the hikers' parking area, to your right, about 100 yards before the campground. Be sure to display your Adventure Pass on your parked vehicle.

The signed trailhead is across the road, directly opposite the entrance to the parking area. Follow the narrow pathway as it switchbacks south up through a forest of oaks, manzanitas, and big-cone Douglas-firs 0.5 mile to a junction, and then turn right. Continue along the trail, climbing steadily eastward with the broad canyon of Big Rock Creek visible to your left, past a variety of interesting rock formations created by the fault, and across several small tributary canyons. Three miles from where you started, the trail descends slightly to reach the rock-strewn wash of Dorr Canyon sweeping down from your right. You may lose the trail as you scramble several hundred yards across the canyon bottom, but you should regain it on the other side as it continues up a narrow valley and across another tributary featuring a small waterfall, before finally arriving at 6,565-foot Vincent Gap, 5.5 miles from the trailhead.

Here, you are presented with a wide variety of options. If you're already tired from the climb up, you can rest awhile and return the way you came. If you still have some gas left in your tank, you can cross the highway and take the easy 4-mile round-trip stroll to Big Horn Mine and back (*see* Hike 82) and then return down to the trailhead, a total distance of 15 miles. Or, you can make it a two-day backpack and drop down into the upper East Fork country, spend the night at Mine Gulch Trail Camp (*see* Hike 83), and then continue all the way down to the East Fork Ranger Station (*see* Hike 85)—a very scenic 21.5-mile transit across nearly the entire range. Finally, a very interesting loop trip—admittedly requiring an extensive amount of driving—can be created with a 10-mile car shuttle between Vincent Gap and Islip Saddle, where you can take the South Fork Trail (*see* Hike 70) back down to your other car at South Fork Campground.

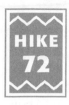

WEST FORK OF THE SAN GABRIEL RIVER, CA 39 TO GLENN TRAIL CAMP, COGSWELL DAM AND RESERVOIR

HIKE 72

HIKE LENGTH: 16 miles round-trip; 800' elevation gain
DIFFICULTY: Strenuous (1 day); moderate (2 days)
SEASON: All year
TOPO MAPS: *Glendora, Azusa*

Features

The mountain watershed of the San Gabriel River can be compared to a colossal live oak, standing squat on a stout trunk, with an erect center limb and long horizontal branches extending outward in both directions. The great branch extending almost straight westward is known to thousands of hikers, campers, and anglers simply as the West Fork.

The West Fork cuts a deep V-shaped trench, separating the front range from the high country to the north. Fed by the waters of numerous tributaries, an all-year stream graces the canyon bowels, shaded much of the way by oaks, alders, maples, and sycamores. Some of the densest chaparral in the range blankets the north slopes of the West Fork, while the steeper south flanks are covered with big-cone Douglas-firs.

Since civilized humans first entered the San Gabriels, the West Fork has been an angler's delight—more so in the past than today. One historian wrote: "The waters of the West Fork were so loaded with fish that in 1892, Frank Bolt, president of the San Gabriel Valley Bank, caught 100 trout in one pool and then became so carried away with his success that he fell in."

This trip leaves CA 39 where it bridges the West Fork and follows the streamside fire road 8 miles up-canyon to Glenn Trail Camp and Cogswell Dam. If you're going all the way, it's best to make the trip a backpack and stay the night at the shady trail camp. Fishing is allowed on the West Fork up to the second bridge; beyond, it's catch-and-release fishing only. No fishing is permitted in Cogswell Reservoir.

Description

Drive up CA 39 to the parking area adjacent to the highway bridge crossing the West Fork, 11.5 miles from Azusa, 1 mile past Rincon

Ranger Station. Be sure to display your Adventure Pass on your parked vehicle.

On the south side of the bridge, pass a locked gate and walk west up the fire road that follows the stream. In a mile you pass the junction of the Bear Creek Trail, leading up into the San Gabriel Wilderness (*see* Hike 74). Just beyond, you cross a bridge to the north bank. Follow it awhile, and then recross the stream and follow the shadier south bank the rest of the way. You pass the rugged portals of Big Mermaids and Little Mermaids Canyons, trailless and inaccessible parts of the San Gabriel Wilderness. (The West Fork here serves as the south boundary of the wilderness.) After 4 miles, the canyon narrows and the sidewalls steepen, with sheer rock cliffs here and there. In 7 miles, you reach Glenn Trail Camp, nestled in a woodsy recess where Glenn Canyon intersects the main stream; here, you'll find stoves and tables. One mile farther is Cogswell Dam and Reservoir, built in the 1930s for flood control.

A short cross-country side trip can be made to the Falls of Glenn Canyon, 0.25 mile up from Glenn Trail Camp. They are three cascades, one right above the other, in the densely wooded canyon. In times of high water, these are the most spectacular falls in the range. Unfortunately, it is not possible to safely view all three at once. With some scrambling and wading, though, you can see the lower fall gushing out of a narrow chute and plunging 30 feet into a deep pool. Do not try to climb the falls or proceed farther; it is unsafe to do so.

Return the way you came.

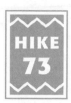

CA 39 TO SMITH MOUNTAIN

HIKE LENGTH: 7 miles round-trip; 1,900' elevation gain
DIFFICULTY: Moderate
SEASON: October–June
TOPO MAP: *Crystal Lake*

Features

At 5,111 feet, Smith Mountain stands tall on the divide separating the North Fork of the San Gabriel River from Bear Creek, smack on the eastern boundary of the rugged San Gabriel Wilderness. From its summit, you get a bird's-eye view over the eastern half of the primitive area, with the deep chasm of Bear Creek right below you. Looming close on the northwest skyline are the rocky battlements of Twin Peaks Ridge, one of the last citadels of bighorn sheep in this range. The sheep were once prevalent in the range; now only a few survivors make a last stand in the most isolated parts of the mountains.

The climb is mostly by trail, but the last 800-foot rise is a steep ridge scramble, partly through brush, to the summit. Wear lug-soled boots.

After a long closure related to the 2002 Curve Fire, CA 39 is once again open and the trail has been reworked and is in good condition. Do it when the weather is cool or cloudy; there is little shade en route.

Description

Drive up CA 39 to the beginning of the Bear Creek Trail, marked by a metal sign, 17 miles from Azusa and 0.25 mile before Coldbrook Camp. Leave your car in the parking area at the trailhead, on the left (west) side of the road. Be sure to display your Adventure Pass on your parked vehicle.

Walk 3 miles up the well-graded Bear Creek Trail to Smith Saddle at the top of the ridge. From the saddle, leave the trail and scramble left (south) directly up the ridge, following traces of a path beaten by climbers. In some spots you must thrash through light brush. You reach the summit in 0.5 mile.

After taking in the superb view, return the same way. Watch your footing during the ridge descent.

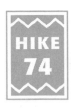

SAN GABRIEL WILDERNESS: CA 39 TO WEST FORK OF THE SAN GABRIEL RIVER, BEAR CREEK

HIKE LENGTH: 10 miles round-trip; 1,800' elevation gain
DIFFICULTY: Moderate–strenuous
SEASON: October–June
TOPO MAPS: *Crystal Lake, Waterman Mountain, Azusa, Glendora*

Features

There are no trails through the San Gabriel Wilderness. There are only trails that touch its outer perimeter and gingerly probe a short distance into its primitive sanctuary. The heart of this wilderness remains as wild as ever. The footpath that penetrates the farthest into the San Gabriel Wilderness is the Bear Creek Trail, which follows the stream 4 miles into the southeastern corner of the region.

The trip begins on a streamside trail that becomes progressively harder to follow and more overgrown until you reach the lonely Upper Bear Creek wilderness campsite. For experienced hikers who don't mind bushwhacking and boulder-hopping, this canyon jaunt is well worth the effort. A delightful stream dances and cascades under tall stands of big-cone Douglas-firs, alders, and oaks, interspaced with open chaparral glades. There are grassy flats where the canyon widens and rock-ribbed corridors where it narrows. Most of all, there is a feel of wildness. Nature reigns here; humans are the intruders. Be aware that there are many, many stream crossings; you *will* get wet, and it is unwise to attempt this hike during times of high water or just after heavy rain.

Once, this was grizzly bear country. In the late 1800s, hunters came in and shot them by the dozen. Pasadena historian Hiram Reid told of one such incident, which resulted in the name for the canyon: "In 1891 or '92 two or three hunters camped in the upper part of this canyon. One night a bear was caught by the hind foot in a heavy steel trap which they had set. He gnawed off his own leg and hobbled away on the bleeding stump, leaving his foot in the trap. The hunters soon discovered this in the morning, and following the bear's trail, shot him. They nailed the entrapped foot up on a tree at their camp, and I saw it there about two years later. From this incident that portion of the West San Gabriel has ever since been called 'Bear Canyon.'"

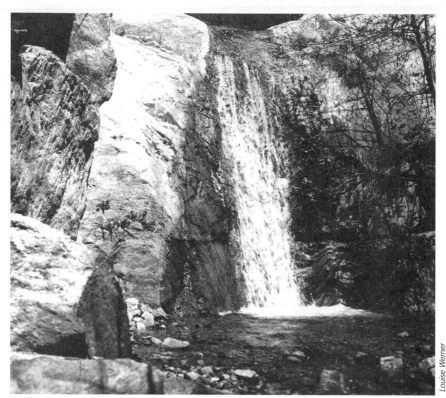

Louise Werner

Falls on Bear Creek, deep in the Bear Canyon Wild Area

Today there are three wilderness campsites along the lower creek, spaced about a mile apart on shady streamside benches. These were once trail camps with stoves and fire rings, but they were so badly vandalized that the US Forest Service removed all the facilities. However, they still make good overnight campsites. The trip can be done in a leisurely fashion, staying the night at one of the wilderness camps, or it can be done strenuously in one long day. Wear lug-soled boots for the many stream crossings and the stretches of boulder-hopping where the trail fades out.

Description
Drive up CA 39 to the junction of the North and West Forks of the San Gabriel River, 11.5 miles from Azusa, 1 mile past Rincon Ranger Station. Be sure to display your Adventure Pass on your parked vehicle.

On the south side of the bridge, pass a locked gate and walk west up the fire road that follows the West Fork streamside. Walk along the road about 1 mile and look for Bear Creek entering the West Fork from the north. Scramble down to the streambed and pick up the trail as it follows the stream up-canyon. This portion of the trail is in relatively good condition and is not difficult to follow. In just over 1 mile, you come to the first campsite, Bear Creek, located in a beautiful grove of oaks and alders. Continuing up the canyon, you come next to West Fork Bear wilderness campsite, shaded by alders, set back a way from the creek. Here, the wild, trailless defile of Bear Creek's West Fork, plunging down from Twin Peaks, adds its waters to the main stream. You may be content with spending the night or turning back here; you've already sampled some of the best canyon scenery in the range.

From here the trail becomes more of a challenge, often disappearing in the brush, requiring frequent boulder-hopping or wading, until you arrive at last at remote Upper Bear Creek wilderness campsite, stretching along the east bank with little shaded flats for sleeping. If you've made it this far, you'll want to stay awhile and savor the solitude of wilderness. Enjoy it, preserve it, and protect it.

Return the way you came. An option, recommended by the author, is to continue east up the trail to Smith Saddle and down to CA 39 (*see* Hike 73). This would require a 6-mile car shuttle and results in a total of 11 miles of hiking.

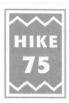

SOLDIER CREEK TRAIL: CA 39 TO LEWIS FALLS

HIKE LENGTH: 1 mile round-trip; 250' elevation gain
DIFFICULTY: Easy
SEASON: All year
TOPO MAP: *Crystal Lake*

Features

Green, woodsy Soldier Creek has been a place of sylvan enchant-ment. Tucked away under high ridges in the upper reaches of the San Gabriel's North Fork, the creek seldom suffers the full glare of sun-light. Its singing waters glide and tumble beneath overarching oaks, sycamores, and alders. In summer, when the surrounding country is hot and dry, the little canyon of Soldier Creek is a damp and verdant oasis. Although the 2002 Curve Fire scorched most of the canyon and the surrounding slopes, the area is recovering nicely and is well worth visiting once again.

The trail is short—only 0.5 mile from the highway crossing to Lewis Falls (named for the late district ranger Anselmo Lewis)—but it makes up in delightful quality what it lacks in length. It is a place to saunter, rest, and contemplate; you will return from it feeling refreshed and revitalized.

Description

Drive up CA 39 to the unmarked Soldier Creek crossing, 2.5 miles above Coldbrook Camp, 19.5 miles from Azusa, and about 100 yards short of highway mileage marker 34.83. Leave the car in any one of the wide spots along the shoulder of the road. Be sure to display your Adventure Pass on your parked vehicle.

Follow the unmarked trail up the right (east) side of the creek, passing a number of privately leased summer cabins. Several of the cabins are little more than stone foundations, due to the Curve Fire. The trail fades out beyond the last cabin, slightly less than 0.5 mile from the highway. Scramble over boulders, crossing and recrossing the creek for about 200 yards to the small clearing at the bottom of 50-foot-high Lewis Falls.

Return the same way.

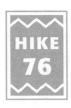

CRYSTAL LAKE TO LITTLE JIMMY SPRING, MOUNT ISLIP

HIKE 76

HIKE LENGTH: 7 miles round-trip; 2,200' elevation gain
DIFFICULTY: Moderate
SEASON: June–October
TOPO MAP: *Crystal Lake*

Features

Mount Islip (pronounced "eye-slip") rises in relative isolation at the west end of the middle high country. From its 8,250-foot summit, ridges descend south to separate Crystal Lake basin from Bear Canyon, west down to Islip Saddle, and east to Windy Gap and the high country beyond. Because its cone-shaped summit stands apart from the other peaks of the mountain backbone, hikers are rewarded with an unusually fine panorama over the heart of the San Gabriels.

The mountain was named for George Islip, an early mountain pioneer who homesteaded in San Gabriel Canyon during the 1880s. In 1909 students from Occidental College, who had a summer cabin at Pine Flats (the old name for Crystal Lake basin), built a huge rock and wood cairn with the name Occidental on top. For many years, this Occidental Monument was a well-known landmark to hikers. In 1927 the US Forest Service removed the old monument to make way for a fire lookout tower, which, in turn, was moved to South Mount Hawkins a decade later. Today a dilapidated old stone cabin, just below the summit, remains as a lone reminder of those days when searching eyes guarded the high country.

Deep in the forest, snug under the east ridge of Mount Islip, is Little Jimmy Spring. Old-timers knew this miniature, trickling watercourse as Gooseberry Spring, for the many wild gooseberry bushes that once surrounded it. It was known by this name when Jim Swinnerton, famed cartoonist, camped nearby in the summer of 1909. Swinnerton's *Little Jimmy* comic strip was enjoyed by Sunday newspaper readers across the nation. Passersby that summer were often rewarded with *Little Jimmy* sketches by the camping cartoonist. Since then, the little spring and nearby campground have been known as Little Jimmy.

This is a circle trip, ascending via the old Windy Gap Trail and descending by the Islip Ridge Trail and Big Cienaga Trail, recently

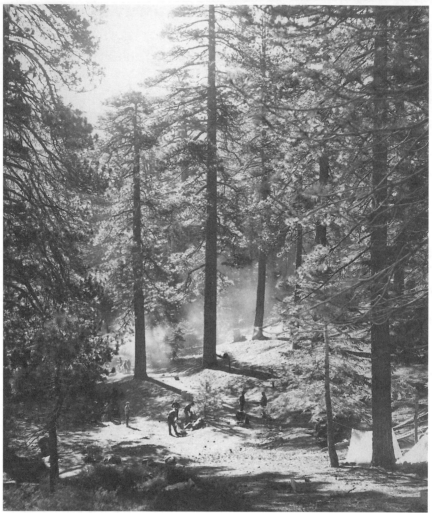

Breakfast smoke—Little Jimmy Trail Camp

cleared and restored by the volunteer San Gabriel Mountain Trail Builders. Sadly, much of the once-verdant pine, cedar, and fir forest that clothed the slopes ringing the Crystal Lake basin was burned away in the 2002 Curve Fire, although scattered groves of evergreens did somehow manage to survive the holocaust.

Description
Drive to the upper (northern) edge of the Crystal Lake Recreation Area, 25 miles from Azusa on CA 39. Park in the large dirt clearing

to your right just before the locked gate. The trailhead is marked by a metal sign across the road from the parking area. The gate at this last 0.5 mile of road is sometimes closed; if so, park back along the road near the café and store and walk to the trailhead. Be sure to display your Adventure Pass on your parked vehicle.

Follow the Windy Gap Trail as it makes a gradual ascent through oaks, pines, and cedars. The trail crosses two switchbacks of the South Mount Hawkins fire road—here, you begin to see the effects of the fire—and reaches a junction with the Big Cienaga Trail. Go right and follow the old trail as it zigzags up the steep slope to Windy Gap, 2 miles. Here, you stand at one of the major trail junctions in the range. Northwest is the trail to Mount Islip; straight ahead a portion of the Pacific Crest Trail leads to Little Jimmy Trail Camp. Follow the latter, passing just above Little Jimmy Spring (unsafe to drink) before reaching the camp itself, 0.3 mile from Windy Gap. Here are stoves, tables, restrooms, and plenty of little shaded flats for overnight campers.

Return to the aforementioned trail junction. Go right and follow the Islip Ridge Trail (signed MT. ISLIP 0.8) as it travels northwest a short distance to another junction (signed, paradoxically, MT. ISLIP 1.2), and then veers southward before gaining Mount Islip's east ridge. The trail then continues west along the ridge a short distance to yet another junction; the sign here says MT. ISLIP 0.1. Turn right and follow the short pathway to the summit. Enjoy the view; it's one of the best in the range. Note the widespread devastation from the Curve Fire along the south-facing slopes; fortunately, the blaze failed to penetrate far past the ridgetop.

After taking in the sights, descend back down to the junction, turn right, and head southwest along Islip's south ridge 1.0 mile, to where you meet the signed Big Cienaga Trail; turn left and follow it northeast, and then east 1.8 miles, through a tree graveyard, to its junction with the Windy Gap Trail. Descend the latter to the roadhead.

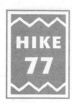

ISLIP SADDLE TO LITTLE JIMMY CAMPGROUND AND MOUNT ISLIP

HIKE LENGTH: 7 miles round-trip; 1,500' elevation gain
DIFFICULTY: Moderate
SEASON: June–October
TOPO MAP: *Crystal Lake*

Features

This is a scenic way to reach Little Jimmy Campground and to climb Mount Islip, starting from Islip Saddle on the Angeles Crest Highway and utilizing a section of the Pacific Crest Trail. The route has far-ranging views out over the desert and is shaded by magnificent Jeffrey and sugar pines much of the way. Thankfully, these north-facing slopes escaped the ravages of the 2002 Curve Fire that so devastated the Crystal Lake basin, just over the ridge to the south.

Description

Drive to Islip Saddle on the Angeles Crest Highway, 41 miles from La Cañada (mileage marker 64). Park in the large clearing to the left (north) of the highway. Be sure to display your Adventure Pass on your parked vehicle.

Cross the highway and pick up the Pacific Crest Trail leading east. Follow the well-graded trail as it climbs through chaparral, and then into pines, to Little Jimmy Campground, 2.5 miles. The campground is an ideal stop for overnight backpackers, located in a secluded little forest shallow, with stoves and restrooms.

A sign near the west end of the campground points the way to Mount Islip. The trail switchbacks 0.5 mile up to the east ridge, and then follows the Islip Ridge Trail, as in Hike 76, to the summit. Return by the same route.

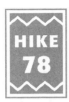

MIDDLE HIGH COUNTRY: CRYSTAL LAKE TO WINDY GAP, MOUNT HAWKINS, THROOP PEAK, MOUNT BADEN–POWELL

HIKE 78

HIKE LENGTH: 17 miles round-trip; 3,300' elevation gain
DIFFICULTY: Strenuous
SEASON: June–October
TOPO MAP: *Crystal Lake*

Features

The middle high country—so named because of its central location along the main backbone of the San Gabriels—rises as a long, sinuous rooftop over the many-pronged watershed of the San Gabriel River. Along this divide stands a progression of rounded summits, rising from just over 8,000 feet in the west to over 9,000 feet at its eastern terminus. From west to east, the major high points are Mount Islip, Mount Hawkins, Throop Peak, Mount Burnham, and, finally, 9,399-foot Mount Baden–Powell.

A verdant evergreen forest of cedars, pines, and firs once blanketed these slopes; sadly, the 2002 Curve Fire wiped out most of the trees on the south-facing side, leaving a graveyard of stunted, blackened hulks. Fortunately, in most places the fire did not succeed in cresting the ridge onto the north slope, leaving the evergreen monarchs here intact.

This trail trip climbs around or over all of these summits, save Islip (and you can also surmount this peak with a short detour), as it traverses almost the length of the backbone. The trail is long, with few level stretches, but it is well maintained and easy to follow. This is delightful summer or fall hiking country. The high mountain breeze is cool and refreshing. The chaparral is knee-high and in clumps, not smothering the terrain as it does on lower slopes. Over near Baden–Powell, on wind-buffeted ridges, are a handful of gnarled, weather-battered limber pines, hardy relics of a bygone age, found only on a handful of our highest summits.

Description

Drive to the upper (northern) edge of the Crystal Lake Recreation Area, 25 miles from Azusa on CA 39. Park in the large dirt clearing to your right just before the locked gate. Sometimes, the gate to this road is closed 0.5 mile prior to the parking lot; in that case, park along the road near the café and store, and then walk in to the trail-head. Be sure to display your Adventure Pass on your parked vehicle.

The beginning of the trail is marked by a metal sign indicating WINDY GAP TRAIL. Follow the trail as it ascends gradually through oaks, pines, and cedars. The trail crosses two switchbacks of the South Hawkins Lookout fire road and zigzags steeply through a forest of charred stumps up the mountain slope to Windy Gap. Here is a major trail junction—left to Little Jimmy and Mount Islip (*see* Hike 76), right to Baden–Powell. Turn right (east), and follow the trail as it climbs steadily along the north slope of the main divide. As you top 8,400 feet, the forest—where it was not burned away in the fire—changes from predominately Jeffrey pines to lodgepole pines. Two miles from Windy Gap, just below Mount Hawkins, a side trail drops 240 feet in 0.5 mile to secluded Lily Spring, the only water en route (purify before drinking). The main trail contours along the northwest slope of Hawkins (250 feet up to the summit, a short but steep scramble), drops to a saddle, and climbs the southwest ridge of Throop before traversing around the southeast side of the peak (again, just below the top, which lies a short distance away up a climbers' path), and turns eastward toward Mount Baden–Powell, now looming massively on the skyline.

From here, you go down across another saddle, around the north side of a forested slight bump known as Mount Burnham, to still another saddle and around one more unnamed welt, and finally begin the climb of Baden–Powell. As you rise above 9,000 feet, the forest thins and you pass several ancient limber pines. Just north of the top, you intersect the Baden–Powell summit trail; from here, walk up two short switchbacks and you're there. On the nearly bald crown are a Boy Scout monument (*see* Hike 81), a metal register, and a weathered flagpole. The view is well worth the long trip: Old Baldy dominates the eastern skyline beyond the yawning chasm of the East Fork; to the south, progressively lower ridgelines disappear into haze; westward is an end-on perspective of the middle high country you've just traversed; and northward sprawls the drab emptiness of the Mojave Desert.

Return the same way, or if you can talk someone into driving around to the Angeles Crest Highway, you can take the short trail down to Vincent Gap (*see* Hike 81). This would shorten the 17-mile round-trip to 12.5 miles.

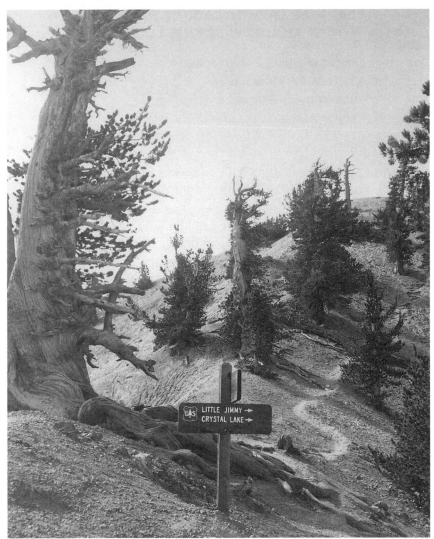

Limber pines on Mount Baden–Powell

Another alternative is to start and finish on the Angeles Crest Highway. Drive to Islip Saddle and follow the Pacific Crest Trail to Little Jimmy Campground (*see* Hike 77). Then continue on the PCT past Windy Gap on the trail described previously. Return the same way. This alternative is the same total hiking distance, but it requires 800 feet fewer elevation gain.

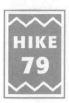

CRYSTAL LAKE TO MOUNT HAWKINS AND SOUTH MOUNT HAWKINS LOOKOUT

HIKE LENGTH: 12 miles round-trip; 2,800' elevation gain
DIFFICULTY: Moderate
SEASON: June–October
TOPO MAP: *Crystal Lake*

HIKE 79

Features

There was never a gal like Nellie Hawkins, a beautiful waitress at "Doc" Beatty's popular Squirrel Inn, high up the North Fork of San Gabriel Canyon where Coldbrook Campground lies today. From 1901 to about 1907, Miss Hawkins charmed and attracted miners, hunters, and campers—just about every mountain man for miles around. Nellie is long gone now, and the doors of Squirrel Inn have been closed for many decades, but the popular waitress will never be forgotten. Her name is eternally transfixed on two summits above Crystal Lake basin, and two other high points along the same ridge honor her informally. The two officially named peaks are Mount Hawkins and South Mount Hawkins; the two bumps on the ridge between are known to hikers as Middle Hawkins and, facetiously, Sadie Hawkins.

This circle trip climbs over or around all four of Nellie's namesakes in covering the high country northeast and east of Crystal Lake. The highlight of the trip is following the new trail, built by Charles Jones and his San Gabriel Trailbuilders, along the ridge between Mount Hawkins and South Hawkins Lookout road, with spectacular views both ways—into the Crystal Lake basin to the west and across the wild, trailless Iron Fork country to the east.

Except for the short scramble up Mount Hawkins, the trip is all on trail or fire road.

The Curve Fire of September 2002 devastated the slopes around South Mount Hawkins and destroyed the historic South Hawkins Lookout Tower. Most of the descent via fire road from the lookout site to Crystal Lake Campground is through badly burned forest that will require years to recover.

Description

Drive to the upper (northern) edge of the Crystal Lake Recreation Area, 25 miles from Azusa on CA 39. Park in the large dirt clearing to your right just before the locked gate. You may find the gate before

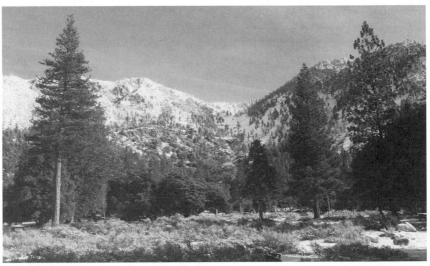

Crystal Lake area

the last 0.5 mile of this road closed; in that case, you will need to park back along the road near the café and store, and hike in to the trailhead. Be sure to display your Adventure Pass on your parked vehicle.

The trailhead is marked by a metal sign across the road from the parking area. Follow the Windy Gap Trail as it makes a gradual ascent through oaks, pines, and cedars. The trail crosses two switchbacks of the South Mount Hawkins fire road and reaches a junction with the Big Cienaga Trail. Go right and follow the old trail as it zigzags up the steep slope to Windy Gap, 2 miles.

At the gap, turn right (east) and follow the Pacific Crest Trail as it climbs steadily toward Mount Hawkins. Continue on the trail as it traverses along the northwest slope of Mount Hawkins. The easiest route to the summit lies along the northeast spur, so you are better off to stay on the trail just past the peak, and then double back and up.

Return to the Pacific Crest Trail and backtrack west about 0.25 mile to the junction with the Hawkins Trail. Turn left (south) and follow the trail down the ridge, around the intervening bumps known to hikers as Middle Hawkins and Sadie Hawkins, until you meet the fire road. Follow the latter 0.3 mile up to the site of South Hawkins Lookout tower.

Descend the road down the burned west slope to Crystal Lake Campground, 5 miles.

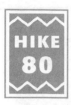

DAWSON SADDLE TO THROOP PEAK

HIKE LENGTH: 4.5 miles round-trip; 1,200' elevation gain
DIFFICULTY: Moderate
SEASON: June–October
TOPO MAP: *Crystal Lake*

Features

The Angeles Crest Highway winds through the heart of the San Gabriels like an elongated snake, reaching its highest point at the 7,901-foot Dawson Saddle. From this saddle, a prominent ridge ascends southward, reaching the crest at Throop Peak (9,138') (pronounced "troop" but named for Amos G. Throop [1811–1894], founder of California Institute of Technology).

A rebuilt trail climbs this ridge and then contours around the north slope of Throop Peak to a junction with the Pacific Crest Trail just east of the summit ridge. It passes through an open forest of Jeffrey pines, white firs, and, higher up, lodgepole pines. Most of the route offers wide-ranging views of the north high country and the desert far below.

This trip, climbing the rebuilt trail to the Pacific Crest Trail and then ascending the south slope of Throop Peak to the summit, is one of the best in the San Gabriel high country. Do it on a warm summer or an early fall day, when panoramas are far-reaching and the crisp high-mountain air is refreshing and invigorating.

Description

Drive to Dawson Saddle on the Angles Crest Highway, 9.5 miles from Big Pines. This section of the highway—between Islip Saddle and Vincent Gap—is normally not plowed in winter and is closed until April or May. Check with the US Forest Service to see if it's open. Park in the large clearing north of the road. Be sure to display your Adventure Pass on your parked vehicle.

The old trail switchbacks up the ridge directly across the highway from the Dawson Saddle parking area. The new route begins about 150 yards down the highway to the east. Take either trail; they join atop the ridge in 0.25 mile. You walk through an open pine forest, first atop the ridge and then along the east slope, gently climbing southward. In 1.5 miles, the old and new trails part company. The old route goes right and climbs steeply up the ridge to Throop's summit;

you go left on the new trail as it contours, and then climbs around the north slope of Throop Peak to a signed junction with the Pacific Crest Trail, 2 miles from the start. Turn right and follow the PCT 0.25 mile to a climbers' path on the south side of the peak. Follow this path to the summit—it's steep but easygoing.

You have a choice of routes on the return. You can, of course, descend the same way you came up. Or you can take the old but well-trod route that drops, steeply at first, down the northwest ridge, joining the new trail in 0.5 mile. Other options, requiring car shuttles, are to follow the PCT east to Mount Baden–Powell and down to Vincent Gap (*see* Hike 81), or go west on the PCT down to Windy Gap, Little Jimmy Campground, and Islip Saddle (*see* Hike 77).

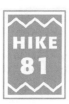

VINCENT GAP TO MOUNT BADEN–POWELL

HIKE LENGTH: 8 miles round-trip; 2,800' elevation gain
DIFFICULTY: Moderate
SEASON: June–October
TOPO MAP: *Crystal Lake*

Features

Next to Old Baldy, Mount Baden–Powell (9,399') is probably the most popular mountain climb in the San Gabriels. A superb trail climbs directly up the northeast ridge to the summit in 41 switchbacks (the most of any trail in the range), with panoramic views north over the Mojave Desert and southeast into the deep chasm of the East Fork of the San Gabriel River. The trip is a living demonstration of how the forest changes with altitude: from oaks and Jeffrey pines, through white firs, into lodgepole pines, and finally a scattering of ancient, gnarled limber pines clinging to bare slopes above 9,000 feet.

For many years, the peak was known as North Baldy. In 1931 the US Forest Service and U.S. Board on Geographic Names sanctioned a request by C. J. Carlson, Western Regional Boy Scout Director, to rename the peak after Lord Robert Stevenson Smyth Baden–Powell (1847–1941), a British Army officer who founded the Boy Scout

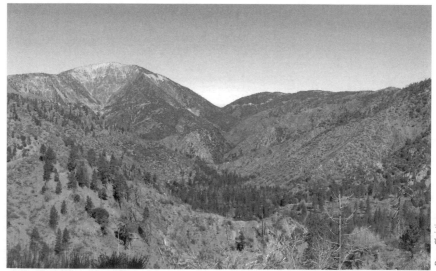

Mount Baden–Powell

movement in 1907. The official dedication of the new name took place on May 30, 1931, when a large party of Los Angeles–area Boy Scouts erected a plaque and flagpole on the summit. Three years later, Civilian Conservation Corps workers constructed the present 4-mile zigzagging trail from Vincent Gap to the top.

For the next 26 years, the peak was all but forgotten by the Scouts; the plaque disappeared and the flagstaff became bent and rusted. This sad situation was brought to the attention of Michael H. "Wally" Waldron, member of the executive board of the Boy Scouts of America, Los Angeles Area Council. Under Waldron's inspiration, more than 2,000 Boy Scouts took part in a nine-week project to erect a permanent bronze-and-cement monument on the summit. The official rededication took place on September 28, 1957. Since then, Boy Scouts have made an annual Silver Moccasin pilgrimage across the San Gabriels to the peak. On the summit ridge is a grove of 2,000-year-old, weather-bent limber pines, discovered by Angeles National Forest Supervisor Sim Jarvi in 1962. One of the largest specimens is named the Waldron Tree, in honor of the volunteer Scout leader who organized the Boy Scout homage to the mountaintop.

Description
Leave your car at the Vincent Gap parking area on the Angeles Crest Highway, 5.5 miles west of Big Pines. Be sure to display your Adventure Pass on your parked vehicle.

A large wooden sign indicates BADEN-POWELL TRAIL—4 MILES. The trail starts up wooden steps, and then switchbacks upward through a lush forest of oaks and Jeffrey pines, with a scattering of sugar pines and incense cedars also dotting the slopes. It continues climbing steadily up the long northeast ridge of the mountain. At 1.5 miles, an unmarked side trail leads left (southeast) 200 yards to Lamel Spring, which has the only water en route. At about 2 miles, white firs begin to predominate, and shortly beyond that, the first lodgepole pines appear. As the trail tops 8,000 feet, the view opens out to the north, where the tawny expanse of the Mojave Desert fades into distant desert ranges. Now, the forest thins and becomes almost exclusively lodgepole pines, tall and erect. The trail steepens, and the switchbacks shorten.

At 3.5 miles (9,000') the first aged, gnarled limber pines are encountered. A small sign points right (southwest) to a limber pine forest, 300 yards on a side trail. Four switchbacks beyond, the trail

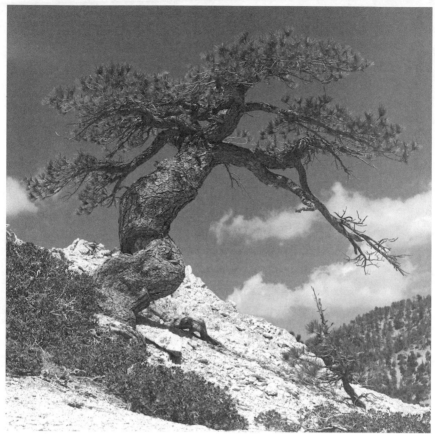

Twisted limber pine near Mount Baden-Powell

abruptly emerges atop the ridge, with spectacular views eastward into the Prairie Fork of the San Gabriel and the gray bulk of Old Baldy on the skyline. Just before the final climb to the summit, the crest trail branches off to the right; its sign indicates 6 miles to Little Jimmy Spring and 9 miles to Crystal Lake. Two more switchbacks, past scattered limber pines and lodgepole pines, and the trail reaches the 9,399-foot summit, with its Boy Scout monument, metal register box (usually full), and flagpole. The panorama is well worth the climb (providing that the lower atmosphere is not clogged with brown murkiness): a vast expanse of mountain, desert, and lowland scenery.

Return the same way.

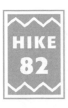

VINCENT GAP TO BIG HORN MINE

HIKE LENGTH: 4 miles round-trip; 500' elevation gain
DIFFICULTY: Easy
SEASON: June–October
TOPO MAPS: *Crystal Lake, Mount San Antonio*

Features

Gold mining—both placer and lode—has played a long and prominent part in the saga of human beings in the San Gabriels. One of the most famous of the lode mines was the Big Horn, perched at 6,900 feet on the rocky east slopes of Mount Baden–Powell. Its weather-battered, crumbling remains are among the most photogenic reminders of the once-feverish mining era in the mountains.

From Vincent Gap, a wide trail (the remains of an old wagon road) contours around the massive east flank of Baden–Powell to the mine ruins. The route, shaded by stands of Jeffrey pines and white firs, offers an almost continuous panorama down into the East Fork of the San Gabriel, with Baldy and its sister peaks rising as a massive backdrop. This is an ideal trip for both the history buff and the photographer.

It was mountain man Charles "Tom" Vincent, a fugitive whose real name was Charles Vincent Daugherty, who discovered the Big Horn in 1894—the climax of a multiyear search for the lode that fed the rich placers of the East Fork. Vincent, a prospector and hunter who lived from about 1870 until 1926 in a crude log cabin high in Vincent Gulch, sold the mine to a group of investors, who spent a fortune to develop it. Thousands of feet of tunnels were bored, and heavy equipment was laboriously hauled in. For slightly more than a decade, the Big Horn prospered. The California Division of Mines reported a yield of nearly $40,000 in gold 1904–1906. But, as with all San Gabriel mining ventures, the veins petered out and the effort was abandoned.

Description

Leave your car at the Vincent Gap parking area on the Angeles Crest Highway, 5.5 miles west of Big Pines. Be sure to display you Adventure Pass on your parked vehicle.

The trail, distinctive but unmarked, leaves the Vincent Gap par ing area, drops about 60 feet, and begins to contour southeast aro the mountain. Much of it is shaded by tall Jeffrey pines and w

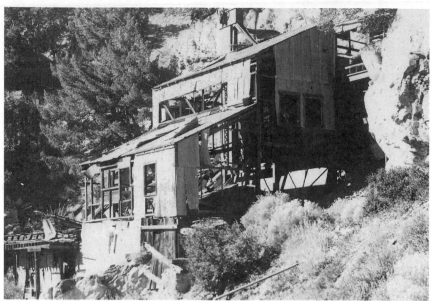

Big Horn Mine stamp mill

firs, an occasional sugar pine rising above the others. The old wagon
road is an easy walk except for a washout near the halfway point that
may trouble beginners and young hikers. Just past the washout, you
pass a small mine tunnel, the beginning of the Big Horn complex. As
you round the massive buttress of Mount Baden–Powell, the deep
gorge of the East Fork, the San Gabriel River, and its tributary canyons come into full view; beyond, there looms the grayish mass of
Old Baldy. The trail rises about 300 feet to top a ridge and passes the
foundations of mine buildings. As you round a bend, the old stamp
mill comes suddenly into view, clinging to the precipitous, rocky
hillside. This is Big Horn Mine, and here the broad trail ends. The
main tunnel is just behind and above the mill building; it extends
several hundred feet into the mountain, is usually wet, and is unsafe
to explore beyond the entrance. An old footpath, narrow and partly
overgrown, continues about 0.5 mile farther around the mountain,
passing several small prospects. The big mill building is dilapidated
and dangerous to enter, as a NO TRESPASSING sign indicates. But
don't be disappointed; the views from trail's end of the huge mill, as
well as views out over the gorge of the East Fork to Old Baldy, are
well worth the trip.

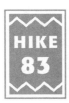

VINCENT GAP VIA VINCENT GULCH TO PRAIRIE FORK, SHEEP MOUNTAIN WILDERNESS, EAST FORK OF SAN GABRIEL RIVER

HIKE LENGTH: 8 miles round-trip; 2,000' elevation gain and loss
DIFFICULTY: Moderate
SEASON: May–October
TOPO MAPS: *Crystal Lake, Mount San Antonio*

Features

This scenic hike is the best way to reach the upper East Fork country. You leave the Angeles Crest Highway at Vincent Gap and descend the broad sloping V of Vincent Gulch 3 miles to the great bend, where the East Fork's main channel elbows east and becomes Prairie Fork. Nearby is Mine Gulch Trail Camp for overnight visitors. This trip is a favorite of anglers; some fine trout swim in this cold mountain stream. Remember that this is an "upside-down" hike—all uphill on the return.

The upper East Fork country is rich in history as well as scenic attraction. Charles "Tom" Vincent—mountain man, prospector, and hunter of bighorn sheep, grizzly bears, and deer—settled here sometime before 1880. His rustic cabin, high up in Vincent Gulch, was filled with the horns and skulls of game he had shot. Prairie Fork was so named because early settlers herded cattle there to feed on the rich grasses. It is said that two perpetrators of the 1857 Mormon Massacre in Utah built the first cabin in Prairie Fork, settling there to hide from the law. During the early 20th century, gold was recovered from the rock walls of Prairie Fork at the Native Son Mine. The mine's six tunnels have been idle since the early 1920s.

Description

Leave your car at the Vincent Gap parking area on the Angeles Crest Highway, 5.5 miles west of Big Pines. Be sure to display your Adventure Pass on your parked vehicle.

The trail is unmarked and easily confused with the Big Horn Mine footpath (*see* Hike 82). You start out the same, but after about 100 yards you turn left and follow the anglers' path down Vincent Gulch. The trail stays on the right (west) slope for a while, and then crosses the small creek and parallels it close to the east bank for most of the

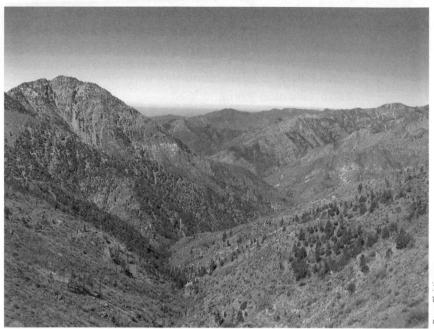

Doug Christiansen

East Fork of the San Gabriel River

remaining distance down. When you reach Prairie Fork, go right (west) a few hundred yards to Mine Gulch Trail Camp, which has stoves and tables.

Return the way you came.

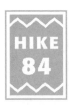

EAST FORK OF THE SAN GABRIEL RIVER, SHEEP MOUNTAIN WILDERNESS, RANGER STATION TO THE NARROWS

HIKE 84

HIKE LENGTH: 10 miles round-trip; 800' elevation gain
DIFFICULTY: Moderate
SEASON: November–June
TOPO MAPS: *Glendora, Crystal Lake, Mount San Antonio*

Features

The saga of the East Fork of the San Gabriel can just about be summed up in one word—*gold*. The precious metal was discovered in the canyon gravels in 1854, and almost overnight the East Fork became a scene of frenzied activity. The only real gold rush town in the San Gabriels, Eldoradoville, sprang up where the East Fork elbows north. It boasted three hotels and a half dozen saloons. Not much more is known about Eldoradoville, for the rustic boomtown was washed away lock, stock, and barrel in the great flood of 1862. Placer gold was exhausted soon thereafter, and prospectors began searching nearby draws and hillsides for promising quartz veins. Their efforts were rewarded, and for the next half century, lode gold was recovered from tunnels and shafts along canyon sides and well up on higher slopes. Place names in the area today commemorate the miners of yesteryear—Heaton Flat, Trogden's, Allison Gulch, and Shoemaker Canyon, to name a few.

The East Fork is quiet now, save for the rush of the stream and the rustling of oak and alder leaves. Prospectors no longer burrow for hidden treasures. But the scars of the gold-mining efforts can be seen almost the length of the chasm. You must look up along canyon slopes to see these aged marks; all evidence of streamside mining activities has long since been erased by the torrential floods that periodically scour the streambed.

This is an interesting trip for more than historical reasons. The scenery here is monumental, on a scale seen nowhere else in the San Gabriels. The gorge of the East Fork cuts deep into the eastern high country, separating such giants of the range as Mount Baden–Powell and Old Baldy. The rise from the floor of The Narrows (2,800') to the top of Iron Mountain (8,007') is 5,200 feet in 1.75 horizontal miles! This is nature in its grandest proportions (at least

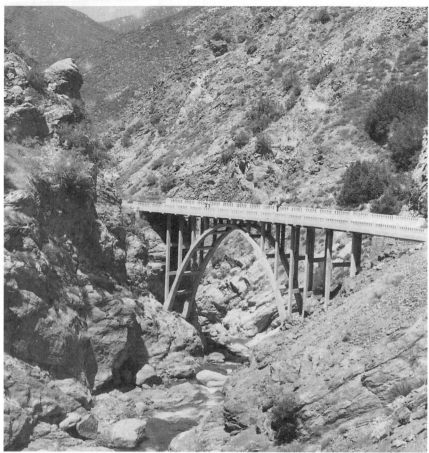

Bridge to Nowhere in the Narrows of the East Fork

by Southern California standards). And there is good trout fishing in the broad stream.

A word of warning: Do not attempt this trip after heavy rains. There are numerous stream crossings en route, and storms turn this usually bubbling creek into a raging torrent that is dangerous, if not impossible, to ford.

Description

From Azusa, drive up the San Gabriel Canyon Road 10 miles, and then turn east on the East Fork Road and continue 8 more miles to the East Fork Ranger Station. Park just below the station. Be sure to display your Adventure Pass on your parked vehicle. Because this hike lies within the Sheep Mountain Wilderness, you must obtain a free permit, either at a self-serve kiosk near the parking lot or at the ranger station.

Walk north along the roadbed that follows the high bench east of the river for 0.5 mile before dropping to the canyon floor. Your trail now follows the river, fording its shallow but rushing waters 14 times. You pass remnants of the old East Fork Road, a paved highway to The Narrows that was destroyed in the great flood of March 1938. In 2 miles you pass under Swan Rock, a towering wall west of the river with the outline of a giant swan etched in gray. When the canyon broadens and curves northwest, climb to your right and follow the old roadbed high above the river. In another 0.5 mile you turn north again, descend 100 feet, and reach a highway bridge seemingly out of place. This is the famous Bridge to Nowhere, the most imposing remnant of the East Fork Road of yesteryear. Cross the bridge and turn right, following a narrow trail that drops into the heart of The Narrows, the most impressive gorge in the Angeles. In 0.25 mile, down to your right just above the tumultuous river, is unimproved Narrows Trail Camp, beckoning you to stay overnight.

Note: The area adjacent to the Bridge to Nowhere is private property. Some mining exploratory work is being done. Hikers are allowed to cross the bridge and continue through the upper Narrows, but please respect private property.

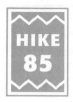

EAST FORK OF THE SAN GABRIEL RIVER, SHEEP MOUNTAIN WILDERNESS, RANGER STATION TO THE NARROWS, IRON FORK, FISH FORK, MINE GULCH, VINCENT GULCH, VINCENT GAP

HIKE LENGTH: 16 miles one way; 4,500' elevation gain
DIFFICULTY: Strenuous
SEASON: November–June
TOPO MAPS: *Glendora, Crystal Lake, Mount San Antonio*

Features

This long canyon trip—best done as an overnight backpack—traverses the middle and upper sections of the East Fork, from the lower ranger station to the junction of Vincent Gulch and Prairie Fork, and then ascends the former to Angeles Crest Highway at Vincent Gap. En route, you pass through some spectacular canyon scenery and visit historic mining areas—most notably Heaton Flat, where Billy Heaton settled and mined in the 1990s; Iron Fork, once the home, vegetable garden, and social meeting place of miner George Trogden; and Mine Gulch, the lair of hunter-miner–mountain man Charles "Tom" Vincent. The mines are gone, but there are some inviting wilderness campsites in the upper canyon.

This trip can be done in one long day if you're in a monumental hurry, but it's much more enjoyable to stay the night at one of the four trail camps, sleeping alongside the stream under stately live oaks and, higher up, pines and firs. A long car shuttle is required between the East Fork Ranger Station and Vincent Gap. (The trip used to finish by climbing eastward from Mine Gulch a short distance to Cabin Flat; however, this section of trail has become overgrown and nearly impassable over the last few years. Additionally, the road from Blue Ridge down into Prairie Fork and Cabin Flat is periodically closed to vehicular traffic in an effort to preserve habitat.)

As an alternative, making the trip easier, you can reverse the trip and go downstream instead of up. The trip should not be done when the water is high; there are upwards of 30 stream crossings en route.

Description

From Azusa, drive up the San Gabriel Canyon Road 10 miles, and then turn east on the East Fork Road and continue 8 more miles to the East Fork Ranger Station. Park just below the station. Be sure to display your Adventure Pass on your parked vehicle. Obtain a free wilderness permit—required for entry into the Sheep Mountain Wilderness—at the self-serve kiosk near the parking lot or at the ranger station.

Leave your other car at the Vincent Gap parking area on the Angeles Crest Highway, 53 miles over the range from La Cañada, or 5.5 miles up from Big Pines on the desert side.

From the East Fork Ranger Station (lower end), proceed up-canyon to The Narrows as described in Hike 84, 5 miles to The Narrows wilderness campsite. It is about 0.75 mile through The Narrows to the Iron Fork wilderness campsite, site of Trogden's. If the water is not too high, you can hike right through The Narrows to Iron Fork. Or you can take the old Pacific Light & Power Trail, built in 1911 when a power plant was projected below The Narrows. To reach the P. L. & P. Trail, descend into the canyon about 0.25 mile south of the Bridge to Nowhere, and pick up the footpath switchbacking up the west side of the gorge. The old trail traverses above The Narrows and then descends to Iron Fork. Iron Fork and Fish Fork wilderness campsites, both a mile farther upstream, make great overnight stop-overs. The old trail between them, high on the west slope, is badly eroded—airy in spots and dangerous—so it is best to walk right up the riverbed unless the water is high. In fact, this section, rather than The Narrows, is the most difficult part of the trip.

Above Fish Fork, the canyon becomes less precipitous. The trail follows the east slope for about 2 miles, and then descends to the broad streambed and continues to the Mine Gulch wilderness camp-site, 5 miles from Fish Fork. Here, three tributaries join to form the main East Fork—Mine Gulch, Vincent Gulch, and Prairie Fork. Follow the trail up Vincent Gulch, 4 miles to Vincent Gap.

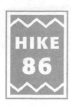

EAST FORK RANGER STATION TO SHEEP MOUNTAIN WILDERNESS, IRON MOUNTAIN

HIKE 86

HIKE LENGTH: 15 miles round-trip; 6,000' elevation gain
DIFFICULTY: Strenuous
SEASON: March–June
TOPO MAPS: *Glendora, Mount Baldy, Mount San Antonio*

Features

Iron Mountain, at 8,007 feet, is by far the least accessible peak in the San Gabriels. It towers as a mighty sentinel at the west end of San Antonio Ridge, standing perpetual guard over the East Fork of the San Gabriel River, whose waters rampage a mile below. No trails approach its isolated summit, and to climb it you must start miles away and thousands of feet below.

East Fork miners knew it as Sheep Mountain, for the large herds of bighorn sheep that once made their home on its rugged flanks. Today Iron Mountain is a last citadel of these "statuesque masters of the arid crags," as author and zoologist A. Starker Leopold described them. Easily disturbed by man, about 250 bighorn sheep remain in the most isolated recesses of the range.

This is a long, extremely strenuous climb for the first 2,500 feet on trail, and the last 3,500 feet up is a trailless, chaparral- and forest-covered ridge. Do it only if you are in excellent physical condition. Wear lug-soled boots and carry two full water bottles. This trip can be dangerous under wintery conditions; the ridge becomes icy and footing can be slippery—definitely not recommended. Someone signing the summit register called this "the mother of all hikes," which indeed it is, at least for the San Gabriels.

Description

From Azusa, drive up San Gabriel Canyon 10 miles, and then turn right (east) and follow the East Fork Road another 8 miles to the East Fork Ranger Station. Park just beyond the station in the large clearing. Be sure to display your Adventure Pass on your parked vehicle. A free wilderness permit is required when entering the Sheep Mountain Wilderness from this trailhead only. You can obtain one from the ranger station or from the self-serve kiosk near the parking lot.

Walk north along the fire road above the East Fork around two bends to the beginning of the Heaton Flat Trail, about 0.2 mile. Turn right

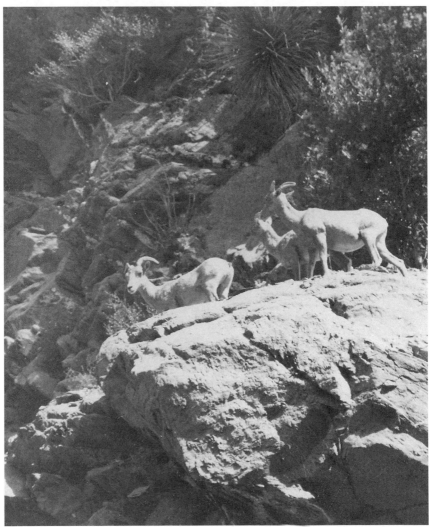

Glen Owens

Nelson bighorn sheep in East Fork

and follow the signed Heaton Flat Trail east to the ridgetop, and then northeast along the ridge to a 4,582-foot saddle, 5 miles from the start. Here, you leave the trail. Climb north, directly up the ridge, following a distinct path forged by climbers over the years. You reach a small saddle at 6,100 feet. Above it, you're climbing in a forest of pines and firs, a great improvement over the thorny chaparral. Continue up the ridge to the 8,007-foot forested summit, where you will find a U.S. Geological Survey benchmark and a register left by Sierra Club climbers.

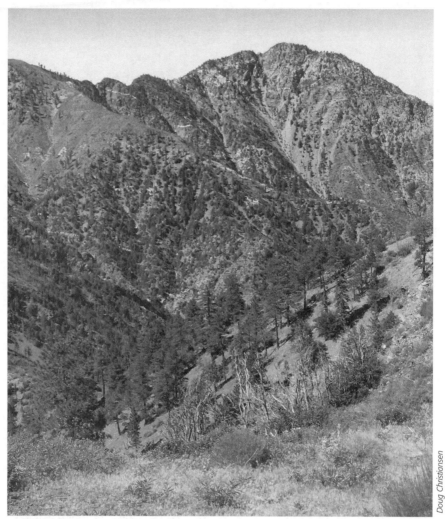

Iron Mountain

Walk a few feet in any direction to enjoy a superb panorama, one of the best in the whole range. The peak falls sharply off in every direction except east, where broken San Antonio Ridge joins Iron Mountain to the Baldy massif. Climbers have reached Iron Mountain via this ridge, either going over the top of Mount Baldy and traversing the entire ridge, or climbing up from Fish Fork (*see* Hike 87). Both of these routes are long, difficult, and dangerous.

Descend the way you came.

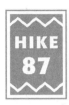

HIKE 87

BLUE RIDGE TO PRAIRIE FORK, PINE MOUNTAIN RIDGE, SHEEP MOUNTAIN WILDERNESS, LITTLE FISH FORK, UPPER FISH FORK

HIKE LENGTH: 9–15 miles round-trip; 1,800' elevation gain
DIFFICULTY: Strenuous
SEASON: June–October
TOPO MAP: *Mount San Antonio*

Features

The rugged, rock-ribbed chasm of the Fish Fork of the San Gabriel River is one of the most isolated and wild recesses in the San Gabriel Mountains. The canyon is wedged tightly between two high mountain ridges—the long hogback of Pine Mountain Ridge on the north and the sawtooth wall of San Antonio Ridge on the south. Looming high over its head is the gray mass of Old Baldy. Melting snows from the great mountain nourish the stream that swishes, tumbles, and somersaults down the chasm. Dotting the slopes and crowding the sheltered recesses are isolated stands of ponderosa pines, white firs, and incense cedars, along with many stumps—the area was logged many years ago. The air is crisp with the chill of elevation.

If you like the high country to yourself, this is the trip for you. In summer, when lines of hikers tramp the more familiar trails out of Crystal Lake and San Antonio Canyon, and crawl over the summits of the Angeles Crest, walk this footpath from Pine Mountain Ridge to Fish Fork to relish the solitude and quiet beauty you find here. At trail's end in Upper Fish Fork is an unimproved camping area, set in a sylvan sanctuary deep in the bowels of the canyon. You may want to spend some time here; it's one of the most isolated haunts in the Angeles.

In recent years, the US Forest Service has periodically closed the road down into Prairie Fork to preserve habitat. Check ahead before attempting this hike. If the road is closed, you must park your car up on Blue Ridge, at Guffy Campground. This adds 6 miles, as well as an 1,800-foot descent and climb to the hike, necessitating an overnight stay in Fish Fork.

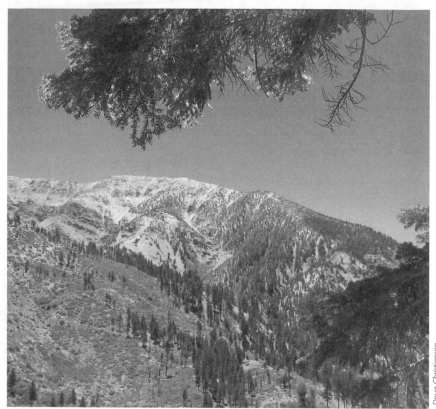

Back side of Mount San Antonio, commonly called Old Baldy

Description

From Big Pines, drive up the Angeles Crest Highway to Blue Ridge, 2 miles. Turn left (east) onto the Blue Ridge Road. It soon turns to dirt, which may be tough going for standard-clearance vehicles. Follow it up and along the ridge, 5.5 miles to Guffy Campground (8,300'), and then down into Prairie Fork, almost to Lupine Campground, 8.5 miles. Just before reaching the campground, turn left and park at the beginning of the Pine Mountain Ridge Road. Be sure to display your Adventure Pass on your parked vehicle.

Walk up the dirt road, passing the Sheep Mountain Wilderness sign (a wilderness permit is *not* required when entering the wilderness from here), and continue up the road, overgrown in spots but passable, to the top of Pine Mountain Ridge, and then left (southeast) down and around the open slope. Here, you are rewarded with superb views down into the heart of East Fork country, with the towering citadel of Iron Mountain dominating the skyline. Keep a sharp lookout for bighorns; they are frequently seen in this area. The old logging road ends and the trail becomes more difficult to follow until you round a ridge and then almost immediately must bear right, to where the trail begins to switchback steeply down the forested slope to Little Fish Fork. Little Fish Fork is an unimproved campsite on a small bench next to the creek, 3.5 miles from the start. Just before reaching the bench is a junction: left is the trail up to Dawson Peak—in poor condition as of this writing and not recommended—and the primitive Blue Ridge–Mount Baldy Trail; the right branch drops down to Fish Fork. Go right. Your trail fords Little Fish Fork, and then drops steeply to Upper Fish Fork, 4.5 miles from the start. There is a delightful wilderness campsite, shaded by tall pines and incense cedars, on a bench just above the rushing stream.

There is no trail up or down Fish Fork; you can follow the bubbling creek a short distance in either direction, but you soon reach rock-ribbed narrows and it is dangerous to continue very far, particularly downstream.

Return the same way—uphill most of the way back.

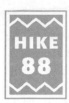

BLUE RIDGE TO PINE MOUNTAIN, SHEEP MOUNTAIN WILDERNESS

HIKE LENGTH: 3.5 miles round-trip; 1,900' elevation gain
DIFFICULTY: Moderate–strenuous
SEASON: June–October
TOPO MAP: *Mount San Antonio*

Features

At 9,648 feet Pine Mountain is the second-highest peak in the San Gabriels, surpassed only by Old Baldy itself. It looms high over the broad swath of the Prairie Fork, razor-sharp ridges plunging nearly vertically into dim forested recesses. This trip, one of the most scenic in the range, is via the old North Backbone or Other Backbone Trail, named as such to distinguish it from the more familiar Devil's Backbone Trail on the south side of Baldy.

Do not be misled by the short distance. This trip packs more bang for the buck per mile than any other hike in the San Gabriels. It is recommended for experienced hikers only and is not for the faint-hearted or those who are bothered by heights. Stout boots are musts and hiking poles are recommended. The North Backbone Trail is extremely hazardous when icy or snow-covered and has claimed several lives over the years. It should not be attempted until the snow melts—as late as June or July in heavy snow years. The trail is easy to follow but primitive, rugged, and strenuous and very steep and loose of footing in places with precipitous drop-offs. Of course, this only heightens the appeal for wilderness lovers—no crowds, no smog, and no screech of brakes, only the high-country wind whispering through pines and firs, the deep blue sky, the solitude, and clear mountain air.

Description

From Big Pines, drive up the Angeles Crest Highway to Blue Ridge, 2 miles. Turn left (east) onto the Blue Ridge Road, which begins as paved but soon turns to dirt (which may be tough going in spots for standard-clearance vehicles). Follow it up and along the ridge, 5.5 miles to the turnoff to Guffy Campground. Pass the campground and continue straight ahead on the main road and in 0.5 mile more bear left at a fork. Continue just over 1.5 miles farther to a small dirt parking lot on the right. A sign here announces the entrance to the Sheep Mountain Wilderness. Be sure to leave your Adventure Pass displayed on your parked car. Note that the gate on this road just past Guffy is sometimes closed; if so, you will need to park your car along the road and walk in to the trailhead, adding a total of 4 miles and a 900-foot elevation gain to the round-trip. A call ahead to the US Forest Service is recommended to verify the status of the road.

The trail descends slightly to a saddle and then begins a no-nonsense climb straight up the ridge to Pine Mountain, which dominates the view ahead. Several loose, talus-covered stretches of trail must be negotiated carefully—hiking poles come in handy here, especially on the return descent. And there are a few short, thought-provoking sections with 1,000-foot drop-offs on either side of the very narrow pathway where special care must be taken.

From the summit, you have a bird's-eye view over this pristine back-side-of-Baldy country as well as Mount San Antonio itself, looming to the south. The view eastward is somewhat blocked by pines; still it's an impressive vantage point—the second highest in the San Gabriels.

After enjoying the view and the bracing high-mountain air, return the way you came. Be especially careful on the way down, for that is when most accidents occur.

An option for adventurous, experienced hikers in top condition is to continue onward. Going south along the North Backbone Trail, this route is a roller coaster ride of a hike that takes you down from Pine Mountain to a saddle, up to the 9,575-foot Dawson Peak, and down again to another saddle, before finally lurching steeply 1,300 feet up the great north buttress of Baldy. This option totals 11 miles round-trip with 4,500 feet of elevation gain, an exhausting but exhilarating day's workout!

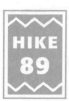

BIG PINES TO BLUE RIDGE

HIKE 89

HIKE LENGTH: 4 miles round-trip; 1,000' elevation gain
DIFFICULTY: Easy
SEASON: June–October
TOPO MAP: *Mount San Antonio*

Features

This is a very pleasant uphill walk on the north slope of Blue Ridge. Your trail starts up through stands of scrub oaks, black oaks, and Jeffrey pines, changing to white firs, sugar pines, and lodgepole pines as you climb over 7,000 feet. Vistas are far-reaching—first, north over Table Mountain to the tawny desert expanse and then, atop Blue Ridge, south into the yawning chasm of the San Gabriel River's East Fork, with Mount Baldy, Iron Mountain, and Mount Baden–Powell as imposing backdrops. This is a hike you should stroll rather than stride, savor rather than gulp. Go slowly and enjoy nature's delights.

Description

Drive to Big Pines on CA 2, 4 miles west of Wrightwood on the north slope of the San Gabriels. Leave your car in the parking area

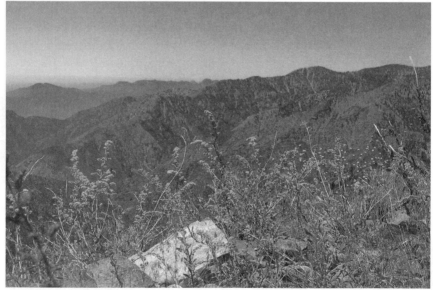

View from Blue Ridge

Doug Christiansen

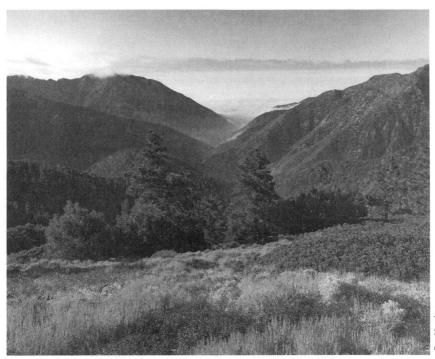

Roy Murphey

Looking down East Fork, San Gabriel Canyon, from Blue Ridge

on the south side of the highway, right across from the Big Pines Information Center. Be sure to display your Adventure Pass on your parked vehicle.

From the parking area, cross the dirt road and descend east about 50 yards to the signed trailhead. (Do not start up the dirt road.) Follow the trail as it climbs around a low ridge, drops to a trickling watercourse, and then steadily climbs through open forest. You cross a dirt road and zigzag higher, with views opening to the north, over Table Mountain to the desert. After 2 miles you reach the top of Blue Ridge and a junction with Forest Road 3N06 and the Pacific Crest Trail. Right across the road is Blue Ridge Public Campground, with tables, stoves, and restrooms. For the best view southward into the deep gorge of the East Fork, walk about 0.25 mile up FR 3N06.

Return the way you came. You may wish to stay the night at Blue Ridge Public Campground.

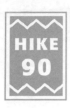

GLENDORA RIDGE ROAD TO SUNSET PEAK

HIKE 90

HIKE LENGTH: 7 miles round-trip; 1,350' elevation gain
DIFFICULTY: Moderate
SEASON: November–June
TOPO MAP: *Mount Baldy*

Features

In winter and early spring, when snow blankets the high peaks of the range and the air is crisp and clear, the ascent of Sunset Peak is a particularly rewarding experience. From the 5,796-foot summit you get a grandstand vista of the great horseshoe ridge—crowned by massive Mount Baldy—that encircles upper San Antonio Canyon. To the northwest, beyond the deep canyons of the East Fork country, looms the line of peaks above Crystal Lake.

It's an easy stroll up the 3.5-mile fire road to the summit, well worth the effort to take in the high-country panorama under winter's glistening mantle.

Description

From the south end of Mt. Baldy Village, turn west up the Glendora Ridge Road. Go over Cow Canyon Saddle to the beginning of Forest Road 2N07, 4.2 miles. Park your car in the small parking area on the left, next to FR 2N07. Be sure to display your Adventure Pass on your parked vehicle.

Proceed past the locked gate up FR 2N07. You ascend at a moderate grade through open chaparral, passing groves of big-cone Douglas-firs and some Jeffrey pines. In 2 miles you pass a junction with the road going down to Cow Canyon Saddle. Continue ahead, up FR 2N07, to a second junction at the ridgetop saddle. Note that the peak you see ahead with several antennae on top is *not* Sunset Peak. Do not continue straight ahead; instead, make a sharp left and follow the spur road as it contours around the north face of the peak to the summit (5,796').

On top, you'll find cement pillars and debris from the fire lookout tower that was once here. After taking in the splendid panorama, descend the way you came. A firebreak drops steeply down the north ridge of the mountain, but this route of descent is not recommended. *Note:* The old route from Cow Canyon Saddle is now blocked by a private property owner.

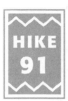

LA VERNE TO MARSHALL CANYON REGIONAL PARK, MARSHALL CANYON LOOP TRAIL

HIKE LENGTH: 5.5 miles; 1,400' elevation gain
DIFFICULTY: Moderate
SEASON: October–May
TOPO MAPS: *Glendora, Mount Baldy*

Features

Between the deep gorges of San Gabriel Canyon to the west and San Antonio Canyon to the east lies a region of low-lying chaparral-coated ridges and meandering oak-shaded canyons. The eastern San Gabriel Valley lies immediately to the south; north is the private San Dimas Experimental Forest. Most of the foothill trails are rather short with modest elevation gains, perfect for beginners. It's ideal country for a stroll on a cool winter or spring afternoon, when the creeks are bubbling, the foothill grasses are a luxuriant deep green, and the hillsides are clothed in wildflowers.

Perhaps the best of these trails lies in Marshall Canyon Regional Park, just above La Verne. The trip described here is mostly on smooth, well-graded dirt road or trail, and passes through a classic Southern California foothill landscape of hillsides and glens.

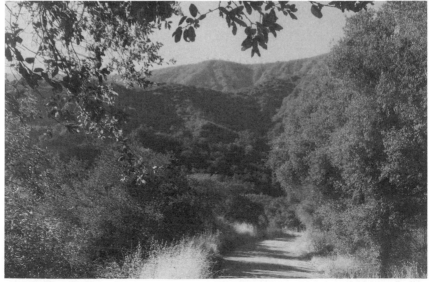

Marshall Canyon

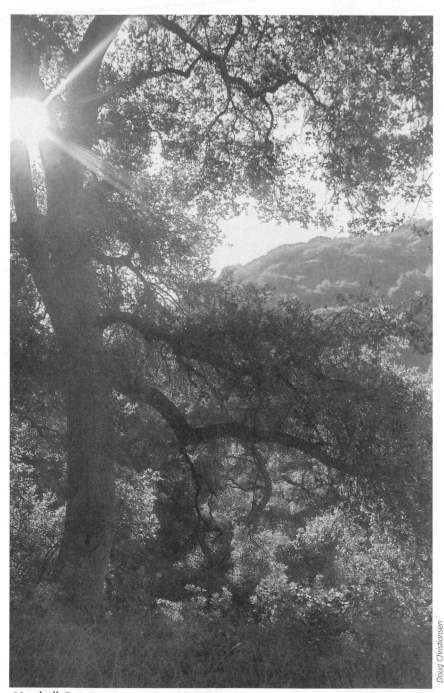

Marshall Canyon

The park is very popular, especially on weekends, so you will likely find yourself sharing the trail with other hikers, mountain bikers, and equestrians (horses have the right-of-way). Although the canyon is a maze of trails and dirt roads, almost all of them eventually wind up back at the canyon entrance, so it's difficult to get truly lost.

An interesting variation on this trip, described below, is to combine this hike up Marshall Canyon with a descent into nearby Claremont Hills Wilderness Park. This option requires a car shuttle.

Description

From I-210 in La Verne, take the Fruit Street exit and proceed north one block to Baseline Road; turn left and in 0.25 mile turn right onto Esperanza Drive. Travel north as the road passes through a residential area and then bends left and becomes Golden Hills Road; a short distance farther, turn right onto Stevens Ranch Road and follow it 1 mile to the entrance to an equestrian center. Just prior to the entrance is a large dirt parking lot on your right. Leave your car here (no Adventure Pass is required).

From the east end of the parking lot, pass through a yellow gate and walk down the signed trail as it descends through chaparral into a small wooded gully and climbs to a junction; turn left. The trail crosses a small stream (water in the rainy season only) and parallels the east fence of the equestrian facility to a fork; veer right and then almost immediately left as the trail continues upstream, shaded by oaks, to a prominent junction (featuring a large bed of poison oak), 1.25 miles from the start. This is the beginning of the loop portion of the trail.

To begin, you can go either direction. Described here is a counter-clockwise hike, so turn right (east) at the junction and continue, under the shade of the live oak forest, across another gully to a signed trail junction. Turn left here—the right fork leads to a dead end— and follow the narrow trail as it begins climbing the east slope of the canyon up to a prominent ridgetop firebreak, affording a panoramic view of the valley to the south. Follow the ridge east, up and over several bumps, to a junction with the Burbank Trail leading up from Claremont, 2.5 miles from the trailhead. Turn left and walk several hundred yards to an overlook featuring the welcome shade of a small pergola and more views of the surrounding foothills and valley. Just past here is another junction, this one leading east down to Claremont via Cobal Canyon. Turn left (west) here, walk around a locked gate, and follow the meandering dirt road back down Marshall Canyon 0.5

mile to a woodsy picnic site under the cover of a live oak grove. This is an excellent spot for a lunch or water break. Continue down the main road for another mile, through alternating stretches of sun-drenched chaparral and shady live oaks, until just past the point where the route bends to the northwest; look here for a junction and turn left. You will immediately see two footpaths branching to the left; take the second and follow it through the forest a short distance to another dirt road. Turn left again and in 100 yards arrive back at the poison oak garden and the completion of the loop. Retrace your steps back to your car.

For an optional one-way trip, from Baseline Road in Claremont, drive north 1.5 miles on Mills Avenue to Claremont Hills Wilderness Park and leave one car here (parking is $3), and the other at the Marshall Canyon Trailhead. Proceed up the route described above until you reach either the Burbank or Cobal Canyon Trail; take your pick. Both routes involve a 2-mile, mostly shadeless descent on fire road down to the Claremont Trailhead and your car, for a total one-way distance of just under 5 miles.

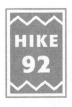

MANKER FLAT TO BALDY NOTCH, DEVIL'S BACKBONE, MOUNT SAN ANTONIO

HIKE LENGTH: 13 miles round-trip; 3,800' elevation gain
DIFFICULTY: Strenuous (moderate by taking ski lift)
SEASON: June–October
TOPO MAPS: *Telegraph Peak, Mount San Antoni*o

Features

St. Anthony of Padua, a 13th-century Franciscan priest and miracle worker, is well represented in Southern California. His name crowns the San Gabriel Mountains—Mount San Antonio. Legend has it that the title was bestowed by the padres of Mission San Gabriel in the 1790s. Early American miners, digging in upper San Antonio Canyon in the 1870s, dubbed the peak an earthier Old Baldy, for its barren, roundish summit. Although the U.S. Board on Geographic Names has decreed Mount San Antonio as official, Old Baldy or Mount Baldy are still favorites of most sightseers and hikers today.

Massive Mount San Antonio—or Old Baldy if you prefer—is the grand climax of the 50-mile backbone of the San Gabriels. No other peak in the range rises to challenge its 10,064-foot elevation. From its summit, you look over a good part of Southern California—an expanse of mountain, desert, and coastal lowland. On those rare days when haze does not muddy the atmosphere, the hiker on its boulder-strewn top can make out the tawny ramparts of the southern High Sierra, 160 miles in the distance.

Old Baldy is a huge mountain, by Southern California standards. Its sprawling gray bulk overwhelms lesser summits and makes up for any lack of sharp relief. Long descending ridges and broad slopes of disintegrating granitic rock drop far down into shadowy canyons. Among the folds of its granite robes are sylvan dells where sparkling streams and waterfalls rush downward, and ferns grow lush in the shade of pines and cedars. Its higher slopes are dotted with lodgepole and limber pines. Some pines stand tall and erect, proud sentinels of the ridgetops; others are bent and gnarled by nature's high-altitude fury, forming grotesque shapes. All contribute to the elegance, order, and beauty of the alpine landscape.

Whoever made the first ascent of Mount San Antonio will probably never be known. Serrano Indians, who knew the great mountain as

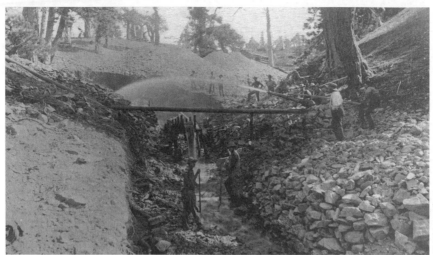

Hydraulic mining at Baldy Notch (circa 1894)

Joat—their word for "snow"—crossed the San Antonio/Lytle Creek Divide (Baldy Notch) centuries before the arrival of the white man, and they may have walked the short distance to the top, although American Indians of that day appear to have had little interest in "conquering" mountain peaks. Perhaps an early miner at the Banks (later Hocumac) Mine just below Baldy Notch scrambled to the summit. The earliest ascent on record was made by Louis Nell and a party of soldiers from the US Army's Wheeler Survey on July 1, 1875.

The first name associated with the peak was that of William B. Dewey, who made the ascent in 1882. Dewey reported seeing no human trail up Baldy, but bears were plentiful and many bear trails contoured the higher slopes of the mountain. Dewey spent most of his life in San Antonio Canyon. In 1886–1888, he served as a mountain guide for Stoddard's Resort, leading many persons to the summit and back. In the summers of 1910–1912, he built and managed, with Mrs. Dewey, the Baldy Summit Inn. Located a mere 80 feet below the top, it was the most unique resort in the West. It consisted of two small stone buildings and several tents securely anchored against a wind that sometimes reached gale force. Saddle horses and mules brought guests up from Camp Baldy (today's Mt. Baldy Village) every day. Fire destroyed most of the camp in 1913, and Dewey never rebuilt it. Dewey made a total of 133 ascents of Mount San Antonio, probably a record even today. The last was in 1936, when he was 71 years old.

Old Baldy is a hiker's delight. The trail is well beaten and easy-graded (except the summit pitch), the thin air is invigorating, and vistas are breathtaking almost the entire distance. During summer and fall weekends, thousands of people, young and old alike, make the ascent. Probably no other western mountain not reached by road is climbed by so many people.

Be alert for (and dress for) changing weather conditions. Summer thunderstorms are a possibility; beat a hasty retreat at the first sign of severe weather. And do not attempt an ascent of the mountain during snow season—well into the warmer months most years—unless you are experienced in and equipped for winter mountaineering.

Description

Drive to almost the upper end of Mount Baldy Road, 15 miles from Claremont. Park on the left (west) side of the divided road 0.5 mile *below* the ski lift parking area, adjacent to the locked gate of the Baldy fire road. Be sure to display your Adventure Pass on your parked vehicle.

Walk past the locked gate and up the road as it winds around the ridge for a good view of San Antonio Falls. The trail then climbs northward, with switchbacks near the top, to Baldy Notch and the top of the ski lift.

From Baldy Notch, follow the broad path east 150 yards to Desert View and a wooden sign pointing left (northwest) toward Mount Baldy. Turn left and proceed up the fire road, switchbacking up a broad slope shaded by Jeffrey and sugar pines, white firs, and incense cedars. The fire road ends at the top of a ski lift just before the razor-backed ridge known, with good reason, as the Devil's Backbone. The trail proceeds along the backbone—people have slipped here, so take care—and climbs around the south slope of Little Baldy through a thinning forest of lodgepole pines, emerges from the trees, and reaches a wind-battered saddle. From here the trail steepens considerably as it ascends nearly bare slopes for the final 400 feet, passing a few stunted limber pines here and there. The top is a gently tapered expanse of boulders, barren of vegetation and commanding the broadest panorama in the San Gabriel Mountains.

Return the way you came. An alternative to make the trip 6 miles with 1,300 feet fewer in elevation is to utilize the ski lift, usually open on summer weekends, for $20 per round-trip.

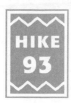

MT. BALDY VILLAGE TO MOUNT SAN ANTONIO VIA BEAR CANYON TRAIL

HIKE LENGTH: 14 miles one way; 5,800' elevation gain
DIFFICULTY: Strenuous
SEASON: June–October
TOPO MAPS: *Mount Baldy, Mount San Antonio, Telegraph Peak*

Features

The great south ridge of Baldy rises in continuous welts from Cow Canyon Saddle to the summit, gaining more than 6,000 feet in elevation in 3 horizontal miles. The ridge begins in dense chaparral, passes through belts of Jeffrey and sugar pines, white firs, and lodgepole pines, and then terminates above timberline. Following the crest of this ridge most of the way, the Bear Canyon, or Old Mount Baldy, Trail (sometimes called the Bear Flat Trail) is one of the most strenuous hikes in the San Gabriels. Its 5,800 feet of elevation gain from Mt. Baldy Village to the top rivals the Iron Mountain hike (*see* Hike 86) for the most of any footpath in the range.

This is the hard way to do Old Baldy, and is only for those in excellent physical condition. Veteran hikers call this a no-nonsense trail—direct, uphill all the way, and in some spots unbelievably steep. Those who complete this all-day trip are guaranteed to be exhausted at the finish.

Years ago, this was the main trail up Baldy. It was built in 1889 by Dr. B. H. Fairchild of Claremont and Fred Dell of Dell's Camp in San Antonio Canyon. The men envisioned a great astronomical observatory on the summit, but it was never built. In ensuing years, parties from Camp Baldy (today's Mt. Baldy Village) would go up the trail on foot or horseback, watch the glorious sunset from the top, and stay the night at William B. Dewey's Baldy Summit Inn (*see* Hike 92), returning the next day. With the extension of the road to the head of San Antonio Canyon and the construction of the Devil's Backbone Trail by the Civilian Conservation Corps in 1935–1936, the old Bear Flat route fell into disuse. This is not a trail for beginners, although it remains easy to follow if you are physically—and temperamentally—so inclined.

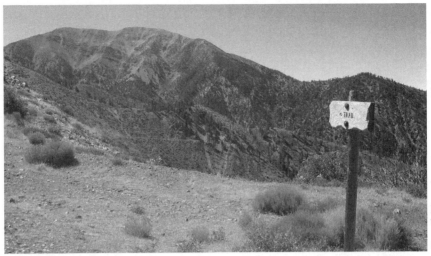

Doug Christiansen

Trail to Mount Baldy

Description

A car shuttle is necessary. Drive one car to the ski lift parking area, 15 miles from Claremont. Return to Mt. Baldy Village with the other car and park on Bear Canyon Road, about 100 yards south of the Mt. Baldy Visitor Center. The largest parking area is at the bottom of Bear Canyon Road, on your right. A small parking area is about 200 yards up the road. Nonresidents are not permitted to drive farther, but hikers are welcome. Be sure to display your Adventure Pass on your parked vehicle.

Proceed on foot up Bear Canyon Road. The end of the road is reached in 0.5 mile, where a wooden sign points to the Bear Flat–Mount Baldy Trail. The trail switchbacks up slopes shaded by live oaks and firs to Bear Flat, a small mountain meadow clothed in a carpet of lush grass, 1.5 miles. Here is the last water en route, so fill both of your water bottles. Above Bear Flat, the trail zigzags very steeply through shadeless chaparral, the most unpleasant part of the trip on a hot day, to the crest of the south ridge. Here, amid cool stands of pines and firs, the view opens to the west, across the deep canyons of the San Gabriel watershed to the Mount Wilson–Strawberry Peak–Charlton Flat country. The trail now ascends the ridgeline, over an extremely steep and loose-footed pitch, known in the old days as Hardscrabble, to The Narrows, a razor-backed saddle at 9,200 feet. After crossing the bare saddle, the route enters an open forest of weather-toughened lodgepole pines, traverses the east slope of West Baldy, emerges above timberline, and climbs finally to the 10,064-foot summit for a top-of-the-world vista.

The descent is via the Devil's Backbone (*see* Hike 92) to Baldy Notch, and then down either the ski lift or the zigzagging fire road to the roadhead.

A satisfying but most exhausting day's walk!

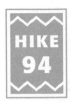

MANKER FLAT TO UPPER SAN ANTONIO CREEK, BALDY BOWL, MOUNT SAN ANTONIO SUMMIT

HIKE 94

HIKE LENGTH: 8.5 miles round-trip; 3,800' elevation gain
DIFFICULTY: Strenuous
SEASON: June–October
TOPO MAP: *Mount San Antonio*

Features

This is the most direct way to Mount Baldy's summit, but it's also the steepest. It's trail all the way, but some sections of the footpath, particularly from Baldy Bowl to the top, are loose and not well maintained. Nevertheless, this is one of the most scenic and historical hikes in the San Gabriels. You pass near the remains of the old Gold Ridge Mine, worked in the 1890s; the Sierra Club's San Antonio Ski Hut; Baldy Bowl, where Southern California skiing was born in the 1930s; and, near the top, the site of Baldy Summit Inn, once the highest trail resort in the range.

You should be in good physical condition, wear lug-soled boots, and tote plenty of water—the only sure source of it is a small stream you cross at the edge of Baldy Bowl, and even this may disappear by summer's end in years of below-average rainfall.

Description

Drive to almost the upper end of Mount Baldy Road, 15 miles from Claremont. Park on the left (west) side of the divided road 0.5 mile *below* the ski lift parking area, adjacent to the locked gate of the Baldy fire road. The hike begins at the gated access road to Baldy Notch, 0.5

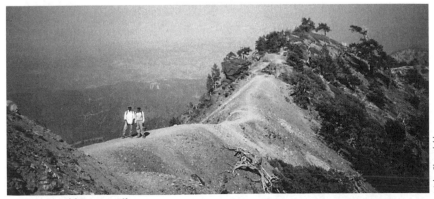

John Skorndahl

Devil's Backbone Trail

mile below the parking area. Be sure not to block access to the gate, and display your Adventure Pass on your parked vehicle.

Walk past the locked gate and up the road, passing a fine view of San Antonio Falls at the first switchback. About 0.3 mile beyond the switchback, look for the Ski Hut Trail that begins steeply on your left. (There is no sign here, so look carefully.) The trail climbs

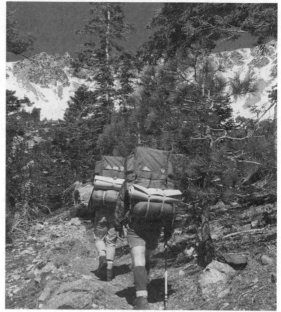

Backpackers at Baldy Bowl

at a steady steep grade up the east slope of upper San Antonio Canyon, through an open forest of Jeffrey and then lodgepole pines. On a sloping bench to your left, 1.25 miles up and about 100 yards off the trail, are the stone foundations of the Gold Ridge Mine, worked in the years 1897–1904. Another steep 0.5 mile gets you to the lower edge of Baldy Bowl. To your right, 50 feet away, is the Sierra Club's San Antonio Ski Hut, built in 1935, burned in 1936, and rebuilt in 1937. You go left as your trail drops down to the trickling headwaters of San Antonio Creek, which has the only sure water en route. The water is icy cold and delicious, but it should be purified before drinking (as should all water in the San Gabriels). The trail, much less distinct now, contours across the lower edge of Baldy Bowl, a skier's delight in winter. Watch your step here; some of the boulders are loose. Beyond, you reenter the lodgepole forest and zigzag very steeply up to Mount Baldy's great southeast ridge. Your footpath ascends the ridgeline, passes just left of some small rock gendarmes, reaches the site of William Dewey's Baldy Summit Inn (open for hardy guests during the summers of 1910–1913), and finally arrives on the broad, barren summit of Mount San Antonio (10,064'), 4.5 steep miles from the start.

Return the same way. Or, with 2.5 miles more walking but much easier going, descend via Devil's Backbone and Baldy Notch (*see* Hike 92).

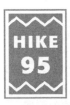

STOCKTON FLAT TO BALDY NOTCH

HIKE LENGTH: 8 miles round-trip; 1,800' elevation gain
DIFFICULTY: Moderate
SEASON: June–October
TOPO MAP: *Telegraph Peak*

Features

Note: Check with the US Forest Service before attempting this hike. The road into Stockton Flat was washed out in a severe rainstorm in 2010 and, as of this writing, is still awaiting repairs.

Stockton Flat lies at the head of Lytle Creek, in a sloping bowl ringed by lofty peaks and ridges. This is the backyard of the San Antonio country, close under the gray mantle of Old Baldy itself. In the shadow of the massive mountain, snow lingers longer than in other parts of the range, providing coolness and moisture for handsome stands of pines and firs.

The flat was named for W. H. Stockton, who filed a timber claim here back in the 1880s. But apparently he did no cutting and never received a patent, and the flat reverted to the national forest. Despite the ravages of a fire several years back, it remains a popular campground and serves as a jumping-off point for this backdoor approach to Mount Baldy.

A steep dirt road, built originally in the 1890s to provide access to the Hocumac gold mine just over the ridge from Baldy Notch, climbs up the back side of the Baldy–Telegraph Ridge to the notch. This hiking trip takes you up this old mountain byway and offers you a number of options. It's a pleasant summer outing, when the air is crisp but not biting, and the open forest offers both shade and sunshine.

Description

From I-15, 16 miles east of Ontario, take the Sierra Avenue off-ramp. Go left (north) and follow Lytle Creek Road to Lytle Creek Village, about 8 miles. Above the village, the road turns to dirt and continues to Stockton Flat, 7 more miles. A high-clearance vehicle such as a pickup truck is recommended, as there are several bad spots that could pose a problem for low-slung standard vehicles. Park outside the locked gate on Stockton Flat. Be sure to display your Adventure Pass on your parked vehicle.

From the flat, walk up the poor dirt road, going left (south) at a junction, and wind steeply up the mountainside above Coldwater Canyon. As you gain elevation, vistas open up to the north and east, across the Lytle Creek and Cajon Pass country. Notice the parallel northwest-southeast orientation of the topography, following the line of California's greatest earthquake fault, the San Andreas. Finally, there is one long switchback, and you round the head of Coldwater Canyon's north fork to Baldy Notch, about 4 miles from the start.

Now you have several options. You can visit the Notch Restaurant, and then return the way you came. You can take the Devil's Backbone Trail to Baldy's summit (*see* Hike 92). You can take the trail south over "the three Ts"—Thunder, Telegraph, and Timber—to Icehouse Saddle, where more options open up (*see* Hike 96). Or, if you can arrange to be picked up in San Antonio Canyon, you can take the ski lift or hike down the fire road to Manker Flat, where you meet the paved road.

This trip offers a different approach to the Mount Baldy country, one that few of the multitude of Baldy hikers ever attempt.

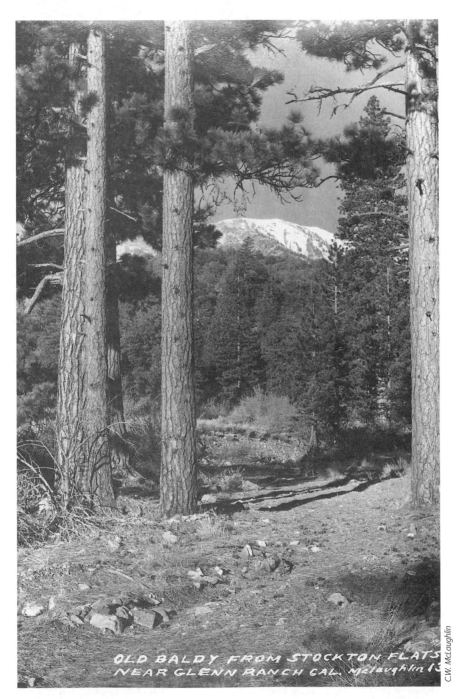

C.W. McLaughlin

Old Baldy from Stockton Flats

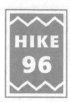

BALDY NOTCH TO THUNDER, TELEGRAPH, TIMBER MOUNTAINS, CUCAMONGA WILDERNESS, ICEHOUSE SADDLE, ICEHOUSE CANYON

HIKE 96

HIKE LENGTH: 10 miles one way;
2,700' elevation gain, 3,400' elevation loss
DIFFICULTY: Moderate or strenuous
SEASON: June–October
TOPO MAPS: *Telegraph Peak, Cucamonga Peak, Mount Baldy*

Features

Between Baldy Notch and Icehouse Saddle, at the head of the great horseshoe ridge that encircles upper San Antonio Canyon, are three summits rising more than 8,000 feet—Thunder Mountain (8,587'), Telegraph Peak (8,985'), and Timber Mountain (8,303'). Mountaineers know these forested knobs as "the three Ts." This trip traverses over *or* around these three summits—depending on whether or not you are a peak bagger—on good trail.

This is ideal summer hiking country. The well-beaten ridge trail zigzags over crests and across saddles, through open stands of pines, firs, and cedars, offering continuous vistas. Snow patches linger in sheltered recesses well into the warmer months. The high mountain air is cool, clear, and clean, with seldom a trace of urban-generated murkiness that clogs lungs at lower elevations. From Telegraph Peak, the climax of the trip, the desert view rivals the one from Baldy. (Telegraph's name dates from the 1890s, when government surveyors installed a heliograph on the summit and signaled to cohorts on Mount Wilson, 22 airline miles away.)

This trip requires a car shuttle and covers a lot of high country, but you get a head start by utilizing the ski lift to Baldy Notch. From there it's 1,100 feet up Telegraph, and then downhill most of the rest of the way to the Icehouse Canyon parking area. For this reason it can be classified as moderate. If you want to do it the other way, add almost 2,000 feet more climbing and consider it strenuous.

Description

Because this trip enters the Cucamonga Wilderness, you'll need to obtain a free permit at the Mt. Baldy Visitor Center. Drive to Icehouse

Canyon parking area, 1.5 miles above Mt. Baldy Village, and leave one car. Drive your other car to the ski lift parking lot at the upper end of San Antonio Canyon Road, 15 miles from Claremont. Be sure to display your Adventure Pass on your parked vehicle.

Ride the ski lift to Baldy Notch (operated weekends and holidays all year). An alternate way to the notch, one that adds 3.5 miles and 1,500-foot gain to the hike, is to walk the fire road from just below the lower end of the ski lift parking area, passing San Antonio Falls.

From Baldy Notch Restaurant, walk east about 150 yards to Desert View, where you pick up the fire road leading southeast up Gold Ridge. Follow the fire road 1.5 miles to the base of a ski run leading to the top of Thunder Mountain. Don't climb directly up the slope; instead, look for a trail branching off to the right. Follow the trail as it traverses and climbs around the south ridge of Thunder Mountain, and then drops 500 feet to a saddle. From here the trail switchbacks steeply 800 feet to the top of Telegraph Peak ridge. Turn left (northeast) and follow the ridgetop 0.2 mile to the summit, 3 miles from Baldy Notch. Return to the main trail and follow it south along the ridge—downhill except where you climb briefly around the west slope of Timber Mountain—to Icehouse Saddle, 2 miles. Then turn right (west) and descend the Icehouse Canyon Trail (*see* Hike 97) to Icehouse Canyon parking area.

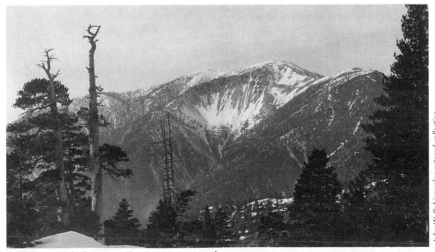

John W. Robinson's postcard collection

Mount Baldy from trail to Ontario Peak

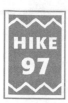

ICEHOUSE CANYON TO ICEHOUSE SADDLE, CUCAMONGA WILDERNESS

HIKE 97

HIKE LENGTH: 7 miles round-trip; 2,600' elevation gain
DIFFICULTY: Moderate
SEASON: June–October
TOPO MAPS: *Mount Baldy, Cucamonga Peak*

Features

Icehouse Canyon is the hikers' gateway to the eastern high country and the Cucamonga Wilderness. Its broad, V-shaped portal leads east from San Antonio Canyon 1.5 miles north of Mt. Baldy Village and climbs 2,600 feet to Icehouse Saddle, a prominent gap on the great Telegraph–Ontario Ridge. The saddle is a major trail junction, with routes leading in four directions.

For hikers of moderate ability, the trip up-canyon to Icehouse Saddle is rewarding. You pass through some of the finest stands of incense cedars in the range, and the ponderosa and sugar pines are healthy and towering. From the saddle you look into the inviting Cucamonga Wilderness country and down over the Lytle Creek drainage.

Legend has it that the magnificent cedar beams for Mission San Gabriel were cut in the canyon and then laboriously dragged down to the lowland by oxen teams. For years it was known as Cedar Canyon (now the name for a tributary of Icehouse Canyon). The present name dates from the 1860s, when an ice plant in the lower canyon supplied ice to valley residents.

The lower reaches of the canyon are dotted with private cabins. Once, there were many more; the big flood of 1938 wreaked havoc here, as it did in other canyons of the range. Today the boulder-strewn floor of Icehouse Canyon bears testimony to nature's torrential fury.

Description

Drive to the Icehouse Canyon parking area, 1.5 miles above Mt. Baldy Village just off Mount Baldy Road. Obtain a free permit, required to enter the Cucamonga Wilderness, at the Mt. Baldy Visitor Center. Be sure to display your Adventure Pass on your parked vehicle.

Walk up the trail that starts just to the right of the parking area. In the first 1.5 miles you pass many private cabins, and the trail climbs gently through a forest of oaks, big-cone Douglas-firs, and incense cedars. You reach a junction. To your left is the Chapman Trail, which climbs in gentle switchbacks to Cedar Glen, 1 mile, and continues on an airy high route along the precipitous north slope of the canyon to a junction with the main Icehouse Canyon Trail, 5 miles from the start. This trip, however, follows the main trail, which continues straight ahead, passes a cluster of cabins, follows the creek another 0.5 mile, and then crosses it. The creek disappears as you climb steadily, under an open forest of pines and incense cedars, and enter Cucamonga Wilderness, marked with a large wooden sign. In 3 miles you reach Columbine Spring, a small seepage of icy-cold water just below the trail. This is the last water en route. Beyond, the trail switchbacks up under a shady canopy of tall pines and firs, passes a junction with the upper end of the Chapman Trail, and reaches Icehouse Saddle, 3.5 miles from the start.

You can take a good look, and then return the way you came. You can turn left (north) and follow the trail that climbs around the west slope of Timber Mountain and over Telegraph Peak, and then drops to Baldy Notch (*see* Hike 96). You can turn hard right (southwest) and take the lateral trail to Kelly's Camp and Ontario Peak (*see* Hike 98). You can go right (southeast) on the trail that contours around the east slopes of Bighorn Peak to Cucamonga Saddle, and then climb the north face of Cucamonga Peak (*see* Hike 99). Or you can drop eastward down the Middle Fork Trail to Lytle Creek (*see* Hike 100).

Whichever option you take, you are sure to travel through some of the finest high country in the range.

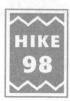

ICEHOUSE CANYON TO ICEHOUSE SADDLE, CUCAMONGA WILDERNESS, KELLY'S CAMP, ONTARIO PEAK

HIKE 98

HIKE LENGTH: 12 miles round-trip; 3,800' elevation gain
DIFFICULTY: Moderate–strenuous
SEASON: June–October
TOPO MAPS: *Mount Baldy, Cucamonga Peak*

Features

From Icehouse Saddle the long, multi-humped Ontario Ridge juts southwestward, standing above 8,000 feet for some 2 miles, separating the San Antonio from the Cucamonga watershed. Blanketing the upper north slopes of the ridge is a lush forest—rather dense in sheltered recesses, thinning out on the crests—of white firs, ponderosa and sugar pines, and, higher up, lodgepole pines.

The Ontario Peak Trail traverses this ridge, staying just on the north side of the crest, from Icehouse Saddle to the 8,693-foot summit. En route it visits Kelly's Camp—established as a mining prospect by John Kelly in 1905, turned into a trail resort by Henry Delker in 1922, and now an unimproved wilderness campsite and one of the best in the eastern high country.

You can do this trip in one day as a rather strenuous up-and-back hike, or you can make it a more leisurely outing by staying the night at Kelly's Camp. If you're camping overnight, you can use the cabin foundations or sack out under the pines. A large campfire ring bespeaks the frequent presence of Boy Scout groups. Just beyond the camp is a small spring, flowing in early season but sometimes drying up in late summer and fall. If it's been a dry year, you should pack all your own water.

Description

Because this trip enters the Cucamonga Wilderness, you'll need to obtain a free permit, available at the Mt. Baldy Visitor Center. Drive to the Icehouse Canyon parking area, 1.5 miles above Mt. Baldy Village just off Mount Baldy Road. Be sure to display your Adventure Pass on your parked vehicle.

Walk up the trail to Icehouse Saddle (*see* Hike 97). From the saddle, take the far-right fork, traveling southwest across the forested slopes. A mile of level and uphill walking through the forest brings

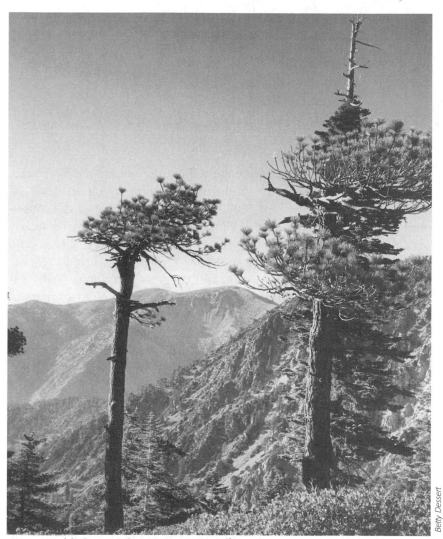

Mount Baldy from Icehouse Canyon Trail

you to Kelly's Camp. Your trail climbs around the left side of the wilderness campsite, and then circles right and climbs to the top of the ridge, intersects the short lateral trail leading left to Bighorn Peak, and turns west. You walk through a lodgepole forest, much of it burned in a 1980 fire, passing just to the right of two false summits, and finally surmount Ontario Peak, 2.5 miles from Icehouse Saddle.

Enjoy the superb view from the top, and then return the same way.

ICEHOUSE CANYON TO ICEHOUSE SADDLE, CUCAMONGA WILDERNESS, CUCAMONGA PEAK

HIKE 99

HIKE LENGTH: 12 miles round-trip; 4,400' elevation gain
DIFFICULTY: Strenuous
SEASON: June–October
TOPO MAPS: *Mount Baldy, Cucamonga Peak*

Features

The Cucamonga Wilderness, enlarged to its present 12,781 acres when Congress passed the California Wilderness Act in 1984, is a high subalpine region of 8,000-foot peaks and deep canyons— pine-forested, precipitous, and relatively isolated. This superb, nearly pristine high country extends from upper Icehouse Canyon and Thunder Mountain ridge eastward some 4 miles to Grizzly Ridge, the upper Middle Fork of Lytle Creek, and rugged Cucamonga Peak. It is the only wilderness in Southern California that encompasses parts of two national forests—Angeles and San Bernardino.

The 8,859-foot Cucamonga Peak is the eastern citadel of the range. Its steep battlements rise abruptly from Cucamonga Saddle on one side and San Sevaine Ridge on the other, offering nothing but discouragement to fainthearted and out-of-condition hikers.

The only easy access to Cucamonga Peak and its surrounding wilderness is via Icehouse Canyon and Saddle. A well-marked trail contours around the east slope of Bighorn Peak and zigzags steeply up the north side of Cucamonga. It's a long hike, but the view from the summit—taking in the eastern end of the range, the San Bernardino Valley, and the mountains beyond—is well worth the effort.

Description

A free permit is required to enter the Cucamonga Wilderness and is available at the Mt. Baldy Visitor Center. Drive to the Icehouse Canyon parking area, 1.5 miles above Mt. Baldy Village, just off Mount Baldy Road. Be sure to display your Adventure Pass on your parked vehicle.

Walk up the trail to Icehouse Saddle (*see* Hike 97). From the saddle, turn right (southeast), passing trails to Ontario Peak (right) and Middle Fork Lytle Creek (left), and follow the trail as it contours through open stands of ponderosa pines and white firs around the east slopes of Bighorn Peak, and gains Cucamonga Saddle. Here, you

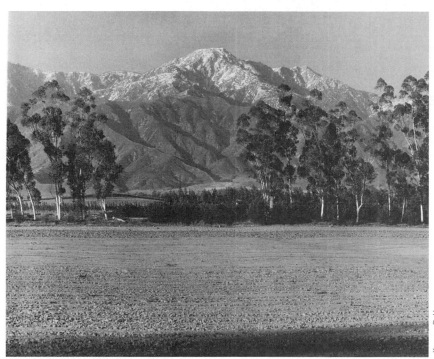

Kenyon DeVore

Cucamonga Peak from the south

can look down into the wild, trailless gorge of Cucamonga Canyon. The trail then switchbacks steeply up the north face of Cucamonga Peak to within 200 feet of the summit and then turns east. The easiest way to the top is to stay on the trail until it gains the east ridge, and then double back up the crest.

Return the same way.

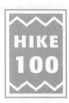

MIDDLE FORK OF LYTLE CREEK TO CUCAMONGA WILDERNESS, ICEHOUSE SADDLE

HIKE LENGTH: 12 miles round-trip; 3,600' elevation gain
DIFFICULTY: Strenuous (1 day); moderate (2 days)
SEASON: June–October
TOPO MAPS: *Telegraph Peak, Cucamonga Peak*

Features

The 12,781-acre Cucamonga Wilderness covers the eastern end of the San Antonio high country, where the mountains are abruptly cut off by the earth-grinding cleaver of the San Andreas Fault. The terrain is as steep and rugged as any in the range. Razor-backed ridges and broken battlements of grayish, decomposing granite plunge downward from Telegraph and Cucamonga Peaks to meet the strange slanting valleys of the great earthquake fault.

This trip takes the eastern approach to the wilderness, climbing up the Middle Fork of Lytle Creek through the heart of the wild area to Icehouse Saddle on its western boundary. Along the way are three wilderness campsites (formerly trail camps) for overnight stay—Stone House, Third Crossing, and Comanche. You start in semiarid chaparral, progress upward through belts of big-cone Douglas-firs and Jeffrey pines, and end up in the cool high country of lodgepole pines and white firs. From Icehouse Saddle, one of the major trail junctions in the range, you are presented with numerous options.

This is not a hike for beginners. Although passable, the trail is steep and primitive in places, with several eroded and exposed sections requiring extra care. Wear a pair of lug-soled boots, and don't do it alone; this is some of the loneliest mountain country in the range.

You stand a good chance of having the canyon all to yourself—99% of hikers who enter the wilderness do so from the more gentle western side, via Icehouse Canyon or Baldy Notch. If you're lucky, you may spot a timid member of the Cucamonga herd of Nelson bighorn sheep—once plentiful but now rare in these mountains. This is one of the few islands of subalpine wilderness left in Southern California—explore it, enjoy it, and protect it.

Description

From I-15, 16 miles east of Ontario, take the Sierra Avenue off-ramp. Go left (north) and follow Lytle Creek Road to its intersection with

Middle Fork Road, 2 miles past the ranger station (where you must stop for a wilderness permit), 7.5 miles from the freeway. Follow the dirt road 1.5 miles to a parking area; beyond here the road may be too rough for a standard-clearance vehicle. If so, park here and walk in, adding 3 miles to the round-trip total. Otherwise, continue another 1.5 miles to the beginning of the Middle Fork Trail, marked by a wooden sign, at the road's end, and park. Be sure to display your Adventure Pass on your parked vehicle.

Walk up the trail as it climbs the north slope above the streambed. In 0.5 mile you round a point and reach a trail junction. Go right, staying high on the slope; the left branch descends to the creek and Stone House wilderness campsite. You pass through stands of live oaks and big-cone Douglas-firs, and reach an open, rocky area where the trail disappears, 2.3 miles from the start. Turn sharply left and cross the creek to Third Crossing wilderness campsite. (This was the third crossing of the Middle Fork via the old trail; now it is the first crossing.) Above Third Crossing Camp, the trail ascends a sloping bench on the left (south) side of the creek, and then zigzags up the slope before leveling off just above the Middle Fork's south branch. There are several sections in this part of the trail that have been nearly washed out, making it the most difficult part of the hike. A pair of hiking poles would be most helpful here. You reach Comanche wilderness campsite, shaded by oaks, cedars, and firs, 4 miles up from the roadhead. You'll probably have Comanche all to yourself; it is one of the most isolated wilderness campsites in the San Gabriels. Don't expect to encounter any Comanches here; those American Indians were natives of the southern Great Plains.

From Comanche campsite, the trail climbs steeply west to the five-way trail junction of Icehouse Saddle, 1.7 more miles.

You have numerous options from Icehouse Saddle. You can return the way you came. You can take the trail west to Kelly's Camp and Ontario Peak (*see* Hike 98). You can go south on the Cucamonga Peak Trail (*see* Hike 99). You can go north over "the three Ts"— Thunder Mountain (8,587'), Telegraph Peak (8,985'), and Timber Mountain (8,303') (*see* Hike 96). Or you can descend Icehouse Canyon to Mount Baldy Road (*see* Hike 97); this will require a long car shuttle.

Summary of Hikes

	HIKE	DIFFICULTY	LENGTH	TYPE
1	County Road N2 to Liebre Mountain	Moderate	6 miles	round-trip
2	Sawmill Mountain Ridge to Bear Canyon	Strenuous	14 miles	round-trip
3	Castaic Creek to Lion Trail Camp	Moderate	17 miles	round-trip backpack
4	Bouquet Canyon to Sierra Pelona	Moderate	7 miles	round-trip
5	Placerita Canyon State Park to Manzanita Mountain	Moderate	8 miles	round-trip
6	Dillon Divide to Dagger Flat	Moderate	6 miles	round-trip
7	Gold Creek to Fascination Spring	Moderate	8 miles	round-trip
8	Alder Creek to Barley Flats	Moderate	7.5 miles	round-trip
9	Big Tujunga to Big Cienaga	Moderate	8 miles	round-trip
10	Big Tujunga to Messenger Flats Campground	Strenuous (1 day); moderate (2 days)	11 miles	one way
11	Big Tujunga to Mount Lukens	Moderate	8 miles	round-trip
12	Big Tujunga to Condor Peak	Strenuous	16 miles	round-trip
13	Angeles Crest Highway to Grizzly Flat	Easy	4.5 miles	round-trip
14	Tujunga to Mount Lukens	Moderate	8 miles	round-trip
15	Altadena to Oakwilde	Moderate	9 miles	round-trip
16	Angeles Crest Highway to Switzer's Picnic Area	Moderate	10.5 miles	one way
17	Switzer's Picnic Area to Arroyo Seco Cascades	Easy	4 miles	round-trip
18	Switzer's Picnic Area to Bear Canyon Trail	Moderate	8 miles	round-trip
19	Millard Canyon to Dawn Mine	Moderate	5 miles	round-trip
20	Millard Canyon to Millard Canyon Falls	Easy	1 mile	round-trip
21	Brown Mountain Loop	Strenuous	12 miles	round-trip
22	Sunset Ridge to Mount Lowe Campground	Strenuous (1 day); moderate (2 days)	11 miles	round-trip
23	Mount Lowe Railway Loop Tour	Moderate	12 miles	round-trip
24	Altadena to Echo Mountain	Moderate	5 miles	round-trip
25	Altadena to Rubio Canyon	Easy	1.5 miles	round-trip
26	Altadena to Henninger Flats	Moderate	5.5 miles	round-trip

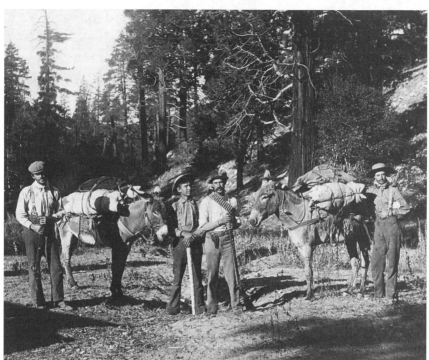

Hunters in Chilao backcountry (circa 1890)

Will Thrall collection

	HIKE	DIFFICULTY	LENGTH	TYPE
27	Mount Wilson Toll Road	Strenuous (uphill); moderate (downhill)	9 miles	one way
28	Altadena to Echo Mountain	Strenuous	13 miles	one way
29	Red Box to Mount Disappointment	Moderate	6 miles	round-trip
30	Eaton Saddle to Mount Lowe	Easy	3 miles	round-trip
31	Eaton Saddle to Mount Lowe Fire Road	Moderate	6 miles	round-trip
32	Eaton Saddle to San Gabriel Peak	Moderate	3.5 miles	round-trip
33	Eaton Saddle to Switzer Campground	Moderate	10 miles	one way
34	Sierra Madre to Jones Peak	Moderate	7 miles	round-trip
35	Josephine Fire Road to Josephine Peak	Moderate	8 miles	round-trip
36	Colby Canyon to Strawberry Peak	Moderate	6 miles	round-trip
37	Red Box to Colby Canyon	Moderate	7 miles	round-trip
38	Red Box to Strawberry Meadow	Moderate	8 miles	round-trip

	HIKE	DIFFICULTY	LENGTH	TYPE
39	Sierra Madre to Orchard Camp	Moderate	7 miles	round-trip
40	Old Mount Wilson Trail	Strenuous (uphill); moderate (downhill)	7 miles	one way
41	Chantry Flat to Sturtevant Falls	Easy	3.75 miles	round-trip
42	Chantry Flat to Spruce Grove Trail Camp	Moderate	8 miles	round-trip
43	Chantry Flat to Big Santa Anita Canyon	Moderate	10 miles	round-trip
44	Chantry Flat to Mount Wilson	Strenuous	7 miles	one way
45	Chantry Flat to Sturtevant Camp and Mount Wilson	Strenuous	8 miles	one way
46	Chantry Flat to West Fork Campground	Strenuous	9 miles	one way
47	Gabrielino National Recreation Trail	Strenuous (2 days); moderate (3–4 days)	28 miles	one way
48	Monrovia Canyon Park to Deer Park	Moderate	6.5 miles	round-trip
49	Duarte to Mount Bliss	Moderate	8.5 miles	round-trip
50	Azusa to Fish Canyon Falls	Easy	4 miles	round-trip
51	Mount Wilson to West Fork Campground	Moderate	9 miles	round-trip
52	Mount Wilson to Devore Trail Camp	Strenuous (1 day); moderate (2 days)	11 miles	round-trip
53	Angeles Crest Highway to West Fork Campground	Moderate	6 miles	round-trip
54	Angeles Forest Highway to Big Tujunga Narrows	Moderate	4 miles	round-trip
55	Mount Gleason Road to Mount Gleason	Moderate	5 miles	round-trip
56	Mill Creek Summit to Mt. Pacifico Campground	Moderate	6 miles	one way
57	Chilao to Devil's Canyon	Moderate	7 miles	round-trip
58	Chilao to Mount Hillyer	Moderate	6 miles	round-trip
59	Three Points to Buckhorn	Strenuous	14 miles	one way
60	Buckhorn to Mount Waterman	Moderate	6 miles	round-trip
61	Cloudburst Summit to Buckhorn Campground	Moderate	6 miles	round-trip
62	Buckhorn Campground to Little Rock Creek	Moderate	5 miles	round-trip
63	Buckhorn to Pleasant View Ridge	Strenuous	14 miles	round-trip
64	Eagles Roost Picnic Area to Little Rock Creek	Moderate	6 miles	round-trip
65	Mount Williamson from Angeles Crest Highway	Moderate	5 miles	round-trip
66	Angeles Crest Highway to Eagles Roost	Strenuous	12 miles	round-trip
67	Burkhart Trail	Moderate	10 miles	round-trip
68	Devil's Punchbowl County Park	Easy	1 mile	loop
69	South Fork Campground to Devil's Punchbowl	Moderate	6 miles	round-trip

	HIKE	DIFFICULTY	LENGTH	TYPE
70	South Fork Trail	Moderate	10 miles	round-trip
71	Manzanita Trail	Moderate	11 miles	round-trip
72	West Fork of the San Gabriel River	Strenuous (1 day); moderate (2 days)	16 miles	round-trip
73	CA 39 to Smith Mountain	Moderate	7 miles	round-trip
74	San Gabriel Wilderness	Moderate to strenuous	10 miles	round-trip
75	Soldier Creek Trail	Easy	1 mile	round-trip
76	Crystal Lake to Mount Islip	Moderate	7 miles	round-trip
77	Islip Saddle to Mount Islip	Moderate	7 miles	round-trip
78	Middle High Country	Strenuous	17 miles	round-trip
79	Crystal Lake to South Mount Hawkins Lookout	Moderate	12 miles	round-trip
80	Dawson Saddle to Throop Peak	Moderate	4.5 miles	round-trip
81	Vincent Gap to Mount Baden–Powell	Moderate	8 miles	round-trip
82	Vincent Gap to Big Horn Mine	Easy	4 miles	round-trip
83	Vincent Gap to East Fork of San Gabriel River	Moderate	8 miles	round-trip
84	East Fork of the San Gabriel River: Ranger Station to The Narrows	Moderate	10 miles	round-trip
85	East Fork of the San Gabriel River: Ranger Station to Vincent Gap	Strenuous	16 miles	one way
86	East Fork Ranger Station to Iron Mountain	Strenuous	15 miles	round-trip
87	Blue Ridge to Upper Fish Fork	Strenuous	9–15 miles	round-trip
88	Blue Ridge to Pine Mountain	Moderate to strenuous	3.5 miles	round-trip
89	Big Pines to Blue Ridge	Easy	4 miles	round-trip
90	Glendora Ridge Road to Sunset Peak	Moderate	7 miles	round-trip
91	La Verne to Marshall Canyon	Moderate	5.5 miles	round-trip
92	Manker Flat to Mount San Antonio	Strenuous (moderate by ski lift)	13 miles	round-trip
93	Mt. Baldy Village to Baldy Notch	Strenuous	14 miles	one way
94	Manker Flat to Mount San Antonio Summit	Strenuous	8.5 miles	round-trip
95	Stockton Flat to Baldy Notch	Moderate	8 miles	round-trip
96	Baldy Notch to Icehouse Canyon	Moderate or strenuous	10 miles	one way
97	Icehouse Canyon to Icehouse Saddle	Moderate	7 miles	round-trip
98	Icehouse Canyon to Ontario Peak	Moderate to strenuous	12 miles	round-trip
99	Icehouse Canyon to Cucamonga Peak	Strenuous	12 miles	round-trip
100	Middle Fork of Lytle Creek to Icehouse Saddle	Strenuous (1 day); moderate (2 days)	12 miles	round-trip

Organized Trail Systems

Silver Moccasin Trail

For Boy Scouts in Southern California, there are few scouting challenges greater than making the Silver Moccasin hike across the heart of the San Gabriel Mountains. The grueling trip was first organized and mapped out by the Los Angeles Area Council of the Boy Scouts of America in 1942. The 53-mile, five-day pilgrimage begins at Chantry Flat, ascends Big Santa Anita Canyon to Newcomb Pass, drops into the West Fork of the San Gabriel River, climbs Shortcut Canyon, crosses the head of Big Tujunga to Charlton Flat, and continues its up-and-down route to Chilao. From here, it closely parallels the Angeles Crest Highway over Cloudburst Summit, down Cooper Canyon and up Little Rock Creek, over the shoulder of Mount Williamson to Islip Saddle, and across the middle high country to climax at the Boy Scout Monument on Mount Baden–Powell, and then down to Vincent Gap, where the hike ends. The entire trip is on good trail—shown in red on the US Forest Service's map of Angeles National Forest. Recommended overnight stays en route are at West Fork Campground, Chilao Campground, Cooper Canyon Trail Camp, and Little Jimmy Trail Camp. Scouts who complete the long ramble receive the coveted Silver Moccasin award.

Pacific Crest Trail

Traversing the crest of the Pacific states from Mexico to Canada, 2,650 miles in length, is the Pacific Crest Trail, the most ambitious footpath in the United States. The proposal to carve this wilderness path from border to border was conceived by Clinton C. Clarke of Pasadena in 1932. He urged the US Forest Service and the National Park Service to knit together and extend the threads of high country footpaths already existing, such as the Oregon Skyline Trail and California's John Muir Trail. Clarke achieved partial success before his death in 1957; he prevailed upon the US Forest Service to call the footpaths in Oregon and Washington by the collective name Pacific Crest Trail System. But not until 1968—when Congress, responding to pressure from outdoorsmen, created the Pacific Crest Trail as a national scenic trail—did active work begin to join together a border-to-border system. The Pacific Crest National Scenic Trail was officially dedicated 25 years later on National Trails Day, June 5, 1993.

In 1977 the last sections of the Pacific Crest Trail through the San Gabriels were completed. Some of the sections—particularly from Mill Creek summit west to Mount Gleason, or east to Pacifico Mountain—make excellent day hikes now detailed in this guidebook. For a full description of the trail, see Wilderness Press's *Pacific Crest Trail: Southern California.*

In brief outline, the PCT route through the San Gabriels, east to west, goes as follows: from I-15 south of Cajon Pass up Lone Pine Canyon, across Blue Ridge to Vincent Gap, up the north slope of Mount Baden–Powell, along the Baden–Powell–Throop ridge past Little Jimmy Trail Camp to Islip Saddle, across the south face of Mount Williamson, down Little Rock Creek, up Cooper Canyon to Cloudburst Summit, across the north slope of Pacifico Mountain, down to Mill Creek Summit, over Mount Gleason, to Messenger Flats, and down to Agua Dulce.

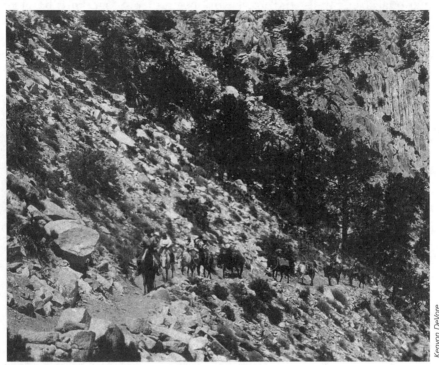

DeVore pack train on the Angeles Crest Trail

Trails that Used to Be

During the Great Hiking Era (approximately 1895–1938), outdoor enthusiasts by the thousands tramped through the San Gabriels. With the building of the Angeles Crest Highway and other paved roads into the mountains, hiking interest declined, and many of these old pathways fell into disuse and disappeared. Others, not preempted by highway, are still in use today.

Below are listed some of the historic trails of yesteryear that have vanished or become virtually impassable.

Tom Sloan Trail: From its construction in 1923 until the demise of Mount Lowe Tavern in 1936, this route joining the tavern with Switzer's in the Arroyo Seco was a busy thoroughfare. Today only parts of the trail are passable. The stretch between the tavern and Tom Sloan Saddle is completely overgrown. The Bear Canyon link is badly eroded by water in many places. Only the last section from the middle Arroyo Seco to Commodore Switzer Trail Camp is in good shape.

Mount Lowe 8: In 1893 Professor Thaddeus S. C. Lowe financed the construction of a network of riding and hiking trails from his recently built White City on Echo Mountain. Most popular was the Mount Lowe 8, via which a traveler could ascend and descend Mount Lowe following a double loop route, recrossing his path just once—near Inspiration Point. Today part of the figure eight is still good trail and part is eroded and overgrown. The readily passable sections—described in this book—are the Castle Canyon, Mount Lowe "East," and Sunset Trails; passable but partly overgrown is the Mount Lowe "West" path.

Lone Tree Trail: Lowe built this steep trail from Rubio Pavilion up the divide between Rubio and Eaton Canyons to Inspiration Point in the 1890s—so named because only one pine tree was passed en route. Today the trail is unmaintained but passable, yet difficult to locate. The lower part into Rubio Canyon is completely gone; the lower terminus is now on the fire road above the Rubio Canyon waterworks.

Cliff Trail: This footpath between Mount Wilson and Mount Lowe Tavern was built in 1919, and for many years the stretch that crossed the south face of San Gabriel Peak was considered the most harrowing in the range. A misstep would send a hiker plunging 200 feet straight down. In 1942 the Mount Lowe Fire Road was blasted across the face, with a tunnel bypassing the sheer part. Hikers walking the fire road today, between Eaton and Markham Saddles, can see the remains of the old Cliff Trail and its handrails traversing the rock face outside the tunnel.

Eaton Canyon Trail: No other canyon in the front range of the San Gabriels can compare with Eaton in ruggedness and inaccessibility. Access into the canyon now is from above, via the Idlehour Trail. Years ago there was a cliff-hanging footpath up the canyon from Eaton Falls near the canyon entrance to Camp Idlehour. Many hikers were injured in falls from this precipitous trail. Today the high fence of the Pasadena Water Department forbids entrance into the lower canyon, and the old path is closed to the public.

Sturtevant Trail: This once heavily trod footpath climbed from Sierra Madre over the ridge into Big Santa Anita and along the west slope to Sturtevant's Camp. The lower third was made obsolete by the construction of the Chantry Flat Road in 1935 and is now eroded and blocked at both ends. The middle and upper stretches from Chantry Flat to Hoegees Trail Camp and on to Sturtevant's are still passable and are described in this book.

Monrovia Peak Trail: This was once a favorite of Big Santa Anita Canyon hikers, going from Fern Lodge up the East Fork to Clamshell Ridge and on to the summit. Today the middle stretch from the East Fork up to the Clamshell fire road is completely overgrown and impassable.

Deer Park–Monrovia Trail: Ben Overturff built this trail from Deer Park Lodge up the long southeast ridge of Monrovia Peak to the summit in 1914–1915. It fell into disrepair when Deer Park was abandoned after the 1938 flood.

Colby Trail: Author Charles Francis Saunders once called Colby Ranch, the hospitable home of Delos, Lillian, and Nellie Colby, "the little Canaan of the Sierra Madre." From the 1890s into the 1920s, this was one of the best-loved trail resorts in the range. The trail from

Switzer's over Strawberry–Josephine Saddle to Colby's, built by "Pa" Colby himself, was trod by hundreds every weekend. Today the trail is passable though bushy, except for the last 0.5 mile into Strawberry Potrero. The US Forest Service is considering reopening it.

Loomis Ranch Trail: Like Colby's, Loomis Ranch was beloved by hikers during the Great Hiking Era. This alder-shaded home of Captain Lester Loomis and his wife, Grace, on Alder Creek west of Chilao, was the most remote of the trail resorts, but the popularity of Mrs. Loomis's chicken dinners and apple dumplings kept it well attended by visitors. Today Loomis Ranch is inaccessible to the public.

Sierra Madre and Antelope Valley Toll Trail: *See* Hike 46.

Angeles Crest Trail: This famous footpath, now preempted by the Angeles Crest Highway, crossed the backbone of the mountains from Chilao to Islip Saddle, and then down the North Fork of the San Gabriel River to Coldwater Camp. A branch went from Islip Saddle down the South Fork of Big Rock Creek to the old Shoemaker Ranger Station. Hunters, anglers, and adventurers traveled it in great numbers from the 1890s into the 1930s. Today parts are gone completely, and other parts parallel the Angeles Crest Highway a few hundred feet above.

Azusa–Camp Rincon Trail: When the San Gabriel River flooded in the old days, travel up the main canyon was virtually impossible. When this happened, visitors to Camp Rincon—a popular resort located where the present Rincon Ranger Station stands—took the high road over the mountains west of the river. Today the lower part of the old pathway is still passable; the upper section has been preempted by the Red Box–Rincon fire road.

Bighorn Ridge–Old Baldy Trail: In the early decades of the 20th century, Weber's Camp in Coldwater Canyon, a tributary of the East Fork of the San Gabriel River, was a popular trail resort. A trail was built from the camp up massive Bighorn Ridge to the summit of Baldy. With the demise of Weber's Camp in the 1920s, the trail was abandoned. It has now virtually disappeared.

San Dimas Canyon Trail: San Dimas Canyon is now part of the San Dimas Experimental Forest, where various types of conifers are tested to determine their suitability to the Southern California mountains. Trails in and around the canyon are closed to the public.

Lookout Mountain Trail: In 1913 the first fire lookout tower in Angeles National Forest was built, atop Lookout Mountain, which is a bump on Baldy's great south ridge. A trail was constructed from Camp Baldy to Bear Flat, and then up to the summit. It became a favorite of Camp Baldy visitors because of the superb panorama available from Lookout Mountain. In 1927 the lookout was moved to nearby Sunset Peak and the trail was abandoned. Today it has disappeared in the chaparral. You can climb Lookout Mountain today from the Glendora Mountain Road at Cow Canyon Saddle, utilizing a narrow trail and the firebreak.

Index